NewHope
FOR PEOPLE WITH
Fibromyalgia

Theresa Foy DiGeronimo, M.Ed.

Foreword and Medical Review by
Joseph E. Scherger, M.D., M.P.H.

PRIMA PUBLISHING

Published by Prima Publishing, Roseville, California. Member of the Crown Publishing Group, a division of Random House, Inc.

PRIMA PUBLISHING and colophon are trademarks of Random House, Inc., registered with the United States Patent and Trademark Office.

All products mentioned in this book are trademarks of their respective companies.

In order to protect their privacy, the names of some individuals cited in this book have been changed.

Interior design by Peri Poloni, Knockout Designs
Illustrations by Laurie Baker-McNeile

Warning—Disclaimer
This book is not intended to provide medical advice and is sold with the understanding that the publisher and the author are not liable for the misconception or misuse of information provided. The author and Random House, Inc., shall have neither liability nor responsibility to any person or entity with respect to any loss, damage, or injury caused or alleged to be caused directly or indirectly by the information contained in this book or the use of any products mentioned. Readers should not use any of the products discussed in this book without the advice of a medical professional.

Library of Congress Cataloging-in-Publication Data
DiGeronimo, Theresa Foy.
   New hope for people with fibromyalgia : your friendly authoritative guide to the latest in traditional and complementary solutions / Theresa Foy DiGeronimo.
      p.   cm. — (New hope series)
   Includes index.
   ISBN 0-7615-2098-8
   1. Fibromyalgia—Popular works. I. Title. II. Series.
RC927.3 .D544 2001
616.7'4—dc21   2001021490

02 03 04 DD 10 9 8 7 6 5 4 3 2
Printed in the United States of America
First Edition

Visit us online at www.primapublishing.com

*To Michael Colon and to all those who have
fibromyalgia and also have hope*

Contents

Foreword by Joseph E. Scherger, M.D., M.P.H.   *vii*

Acknowledgments   *xi*

1. Disease Profile   1

2. Diagnosis   37

3. Medical Treatments   65

4. Exercise and Relaxation Techniques   105

5. The Mind-Body Connection 141

6. Complementary and Alternative Therapies   171

7. Fibromyalgia and Life Relationships 213

8. Fibromyalgia and the Future   251

Appendix: Resource Information   271

Notes   275

Glossary   282

Index   286

Foreword

FIBROMYALGIA IS A common and debilitating condition that impacts the lives of an estimated three to six million people in the United States. Theresa DiGeronimo gives us a sensitive and comprehensive book that will be of tremendous value to people suffering from this condition. As a family physician, I have been treating patients with fibromyalgia since it became more widely recognized in the mid-1980s. As aptly described in this book, there is a wide array of patients who suffer from the generalized pain, fatigue, and other symptoms of fibroymyalgia. There are many theories as to why people develop this condition—these are all well described in this book. DiGeronimo also explains the wide range of treatment options and presents in clear language some of the latest research being done to uncover the secrets of fibromyalgia. This condition remains mysterious in medicine, since no clear biochemical changes have been identified that explain the symptoms of fibromyalgia.

Fibromyalgia is not a "clean" disease like diabetes, precisely classified and precisely treated. My own experience has taught me that fibromyalgia is an illness much like other chronic conditions such as chronic fatigue syndrome, chronic headaches, and irritable bowel syndrome. All of these illnesses must be considered from biological, psychological, social, and spiritual perspectives. Fibromyalgia does have a biological foundation for the pain and other symptoms, but psychological factors play a major role in the severity and chronicity of the disease. And while fibromyalgia often seriously disrupts the family and social environment of those who have it, spiritual connection and hope can have a large impact on recovery or management of its symptoms.

The general causes of all disease in a developed country like the United States can be put into three categories: genetics, lifestyle, and what I call "bad luck," such as acquiring an infection, cancer, or an autoimmune disease. Considering all diseases in the United States, it is estimated that genetics and bad luck each contribute about 25 percent, with lifestyle factors contributing a whopping 50 percent to the underlying cause of disease. These percentages may hold true for patients with fibromyalgia, as well.

My own experience has led me to a theory of this disease consistent with research presented in this book. I have yet to find a patient with fibromyalgia who reports sleeping well. For a variety of reasons, patients with fibromyalgia fall into sleep patterns which are not restful, and they wake up with pain and fatigue. We know that deep sleep is necessary in order for the restorative functions of relaxation to occur in the muscles, and possibly in the neuromuscular junctions (where our nerves meet our muscles). Physical conditioning also has much to do with the restorative health of our neuromuscular junctions. We know today that as many as 40 percent of adults do not get adequate sleep, making insomnia one of the most common conditions in the population. We also know that the majority of Americans are out of shape. Might these two factors alone explain the rising number of patients with fibromyalgia?

I have been prescribing restful sleep and physical conditioning to all of my patients with fibromyalgia, and many recover completely. Of course, the root cause of poor sleep must be identified and treated if possible. Often, fibromyalgia occurs in the young mother who has not slept well since the birth of her baby. Menopause can be disruptive to sleep, and many women in the perimenopausal period develop fibromyalgia. Stresses such as fear, spousal abuse, and other personal problems may play a major role in the lack of deep sleep. Stress reduction can be a pathway to a healthier lifestyle and relief from fibro-myalgia. Some patients do leave this condition behind through lifestyle adjustments that result in better sleep and better physical conditioning.

Theresa DiGeronimo has written a tremendous book based on exhaustive research of the leading experts dealing with this condition. I had the pleasure of talking to her at length about my own experiences. There has been a great lack of public information on this common debilitating condition, but this book should go a long way toward educating people—the first step in treatment.

—Joseph E. Scherger, M.D., M.P.H.
dean, College of Medicine,
Florida State University, Tallahassee

Acknowledgments

A debt of gratitude and thanks is due to all the professionals who willingly shared their expertise to make this book as accurate and up-to-date as possible:

Leslie Aaron, Ph.D., Department of Medicine, General Internal Medicine, Harborview Medical Center, Seattle, WA; Douglas Ashendorf, M.D., Clark, NJ; John Astin, Ph.D., University of Maryland School of Medicine Complementary Program, Baltimore; Robert M. Bennett, M.D., Oregon Health Sciences University, Portland, OR; Laurence Bradley, Ph.D., professor of medicine, Clinical Immunology and Rheumatology, University of Alabama at Birmingham; Leslie Bourne, Ph.D., director, Behavioral Medicine, Fallon Clinic, Worcester, MA; Daniel Clauw, M.D., Georgetown University Medical Center, Washington, D.C.; Brian Clement, Hippocrates Health Institute, West Palm Beach, FL; Doyt Conn, M.D., director of rheumatology, Emory Universtiy Medical School and Grady Hospital, Atlanta, GA; Penny Cowan, executive director, American Chronic Pain Association, Rocklin, CA; Kathleen Duffy, herbalist, Florance, MA; Jennifer Gaddy, N.D., M.Ed., homeopathist, Portland, OR; Barbara Gilbertson, D.O., medical director, Klamath Pain Clinic, Klamath Falls, OR; Rea Gleason, The National Fibromyalgia Research Association (NFRA), Salem, OR; Jane Greer, Ph.D., marriage and family therapist, New York, NY; Ken Guiffre, M.D., Hackensack University Medical Center, Hackensack, NJ; Louella Harris, National Awareness Campaign for Upper Cervical

Care, Lakeland, FL; Clifford Korn, N.C.T.M.B., Windham Health Center, Neuromuscular Therapy, Windham, NH; Kate Lorig, R.N., Dr.PH., Stanford Patient Education Research Center, Palo Alto, CA; Urscia Mahring, D.C., Alexandria, VA; Leslie Nadler, Ph.D., director of behavioral therapy, Pain Care, Long Island, NY; Cameron Preece, Ph.D., Syracuse University, NY; I. Jon Russell, M.D., Department of Medicine/Clinical Immunology, University of Texas, Health Science Center, San Antonio; Joseph E. Scherger, M.D., M.P.H., dean, College of Medicine, Florida State University, Tallahassee; Diane Scheufele, Fallon Clinic, Worcester, MA; Vincent Sferra, D.C., Natural Medicine & Rehabilitation, Bridgewater, NJ; Alec G. Sohmer, Esq., Alec G. Sohmer and Associates, Brockton, MA; Steve Thorson, The Fibromyalgia Network, Tucson, AZ; Dennis C. Turk, Ph.D., John and Emma Bonica Professor of Anesthesiology & Pain Research, Department of Anesthesiology, University of Washington, Seattle; Miryam Ehrlich Williamson, Warwick, MA; Eric Willmarth, Ph.D., director of behavioral medicine, Pain Management Center, Holland Community Hospital, Michigan; and Muhammad B. Yunus, M.D., professor of medicine, University of Illinois College of Medicine, Peoria.

Special thanks to those who shared their personal experiences with fibromyalgia:

Ahmie, Aileen, Angie, Barbara, Bill, Caron, Debby, Donna, Emily, Joanne, Karen, Kathleen, Kathy, Linda, Megan, Mirinda, Paula, Pat, Patrick, Raylene, Sheryl, Stacie, and Sue.

I would also like to thank my helpful and competent editors, Susan Silva, Jamie Miller, and Marjorie Lery.

CHAPTER 1

Disease Profile

IF YOU HAVE fibromyalgia syndrome (FMS), it's possible that many of your friends have never heard of this condition, and perhaps few are true believers. You probably get little sympathy from your boss and coworkers when you miss work because you're "tired." It's hard to get anybody to believe that you could really hurt "all over" all the time. And even some members of your family probably get annoyed watching you lie around resting when you appear perfectly healthy.

There is no doubt that fibromyalgia is not a simple condition and even medical experts are not always in complete agreement about what it is exactly and even what to call it. So, for the record, let's begin with a definition: The Fibromyalgia Network (an educational resource group with over 3,000 subscribers) defines fibromyalgia as "a widespread musculoskeletal pain and fatigue disorder for which the cause is still unknown."[1]

This is a nice and neat definition that may come in handy if someone asks you directly to define your problem, but if you have fibromyalgia, you know that this definition is not the half of it. Although it is a benign condition that causes no known damage to muscles or connective tissue, it is associated with sometimes debilitating symptoms. Fatigue and widespread pain in areas around the neck, shoulders, upper back, lower back, and hip areas are common. Doyt Conn, M.D., director of rheumatology at Emory University School of Medicine and Grady Hospital in Atlanta, Georgia, adds that many people with fibromyalgia also have symptoms of irritable bowel syndrome, headaches, numbness or tingling of the extremities, and extreme sensitivity to touch (to name just a few!).

> *Although it is a benign condition that causes no known damage to muscles or connective tissue, fibromyalgia is associated with sometimes debilitating symptoms.*

Fibromyalgia is additionally difficult to explain because it can either exist as an isolated condition or accompany other conditions. Sometimes another chronic pain problem like arthritis or lupus is present. Other times, fibromyalgia exists along with endocrine conditions, thyroid problems, infectious diseases, or Lyme disease. It often accompanies depression or sleep problems. And to stir up the pot further, some say that no two people who have fibromyalgia have exactly the same symptoms.

It's no wonder that explaining this collection of symptoms to others is one of the very difficult things about having fibromyalgia. In this chapter, we'll take a close look at these symptoms, as well as the history of FMS, the possible causes, the course of the condition, and some people who, like you, are trying to put all these pieces together.

SYMPTOMS

Most people with fibromyalgia take a deep breath before they try to answer what sounds like a simple question: "What are your symptoms?" Although the answer isn't a short easy one, the medical community now agrees that some specific symptoms are definitely signs of fibromyalgia. And other troubles are so commonly experienced by many people with this condition that they, too, are considered telltale symptoms.

Speaking Out

The following quotes are from online fibromyalgia message boards:

- "I live the battle every day. I refuse to let this pain get me down; I'm a gardener and I go out and work in my flowers. It does me a world of good."

- "Once in a while I get down, but I love a battle and boy, do I have one."

- "One of my doctors is still trying to say it's in my head."

- "You're not crazy. You have a very real pain that, unfortunately, is invisible to everyone else."

- "We look like very healthy people . . . so usually we suffer in silence to keep from being labeled as hypochondriacs."

Primary Symptoms

According to Muhammad B. Yunus, M.D., FACP, FACR, a professor of medicine at the University of Illinois College of Medicine, who is renowned for his work with fibromyalgia, the most common and characteristic symptoms of fibromyalgia are these four:

1. Generalized pain

2. Stiffness

3. Fatigue

4. Poor sleep

Let's take a look at these primary symptoms one by one.

Pain

Medical doctors should know to suspect fibromyalgia when a patient comes to them saying, "I hurt all over." This description separates FMS from the many other medical conditions that cause pain in only one or two areas of the body. FMS pain is widespread throughout common sites that include the lower back, neck, the shoulder region, arms, hands, knees, hips, thighs, legs, and feet. Pain may also appear in the jaw or chest. The pain of FMS may occur simultaneously in different parts of the body. It is felt within the muscle, as well as at the joints where ligaments attach muscles to bone. There is often extreme tenderness over many of the locations. These sites of tenderness are called *tender points*.

It's interesting that although pain is the predominant symptom, "pain" is actually hard to describe. Some say the pain is *shooting;* others say *nagging, pricking, deep and aching, radiating, gnawing, stabbing, throbbing, or burning.* And this pain, whatever it is perceived to be, ranges in severity from mild to severe. For some, the pain is consistently annoying, while for others it can be so bad that they cannot perform the simplest of everyday tasks.

Some people with fibromyalgia find that the intensity of the pain changes from day to day or from month to month. When they can't stand the pain any longer, they may make an appointment to see the doctor, yet on the day of the appointment, they feel fine! Many find that certain factors aggravate their pain, such as activity, lack of exercise, extremes of temperature or humidity, anxiety, stress, lack of sleep, and infectious illness.

To say that pain is a symptom of fibromyalgia is a simplistic statement. The location, frequency, and degree of pain all play a role in identifying this complex condition.

Stiffness

About 80 percent of the people with fibromyalgia have chronic stiffness through the muscles and joints of the back, arms, and legs.[2] It's the kind of stiffness that makes you want to stretch out to soothe the discomfort. This stiffness has caused some people with FMS to be misdiagnosed with arthritis. Similar to arthritis, the stiffness of fibromyalgia tends to be especially bad upon waking, will improve during the day, and often come back at night. Stiffness is a symptom of fibromyalgia only when it occurs along with the other known symptoms.

> *F*MS pain is widespread throughout common sites that include the lower back, neck, the shoulder region, arms, hands, knees, hips, thighs, legs, and feet.

Fatigue

Fatigue is not the same as feeling tired. Everyone feels tired once in a while, and it's no big deal. But fatigue is the kind of exhaustion that limits your daily activities. When suffering fatigue, you cannot join in the fun of a party, or sweep the floor, or even take a walk. Comments about fatigue in fibromyalgia chat rooms include these:

"Fatigue ruins my day. It slows me down big time."

"What little I can do takes me five times longer than most."

"Walking and just moving get me tired."

"To do housework I have to do some, sit down, and then do some more."

In some cases fatigue may be experienced as a decrease in muscle endurance—you just can't push the shopping cart or lift a stack of papers. In other cases it may be an overall lack of energy or the feeling of being totally drained of energy—you simply can't get up and go to work. Some people say fatigue is often the most debilitating symptom of fibromyalgia.

Poor Sleep

Ask people with fibromyalgia how they sleep, and they're likely to say, "Terrible!" The vast majority of people with FMS complain of not being able to fall asleep, and once they do they are unable to stay asleep throughout the night. Even if they are able to sleep for a normal period of time, they often awake feeling tired, unrefreshed, or nonrestored. A Canadian researcher has reported that overall as many as 75 percent of people with FMS have sleep disorders.[3] People with FMS report sleep-associated problems such as the following:

- **Lack of deep, delta sleep.** The inability to stay in the deepest stage of sleep (REM sleep) during which dreams occur and the body physically restores itself.

- **Sleep apnea.** A potentially life-threatening problem in which a person stops breathing due to relaxed or excessive tissue blocking the airway.

- **Restless legs syndrome.** A creepy, crawling sensation in the legs that creates an irresistible urge to move them.

It doesn't matter how many hours you spend in bed with your eyes closed; if you suffer sleep disorders, you may not be getting the kind of restorative sleep that would help you manage the other symptoms of fibromyalgia. Indeed, some experts in fibromyalgia believe that the lack of deep sleep may be an underlying cause of FMS in some patients (see chapter 3).

> *If you suffer sleep disorders, you may not be getting the kind of restorative sleep that would help you manage the other symptoms of fibromyalgia.*

Other Common Symptoms

In addition to the common symptoms of generalized pain, stiffness, fatigue, and poor sleep, many people with FMS (but certainly not all) suffer other symptoms as well. These additional symptoms include mental confusion, irritable bowel syndrome, and depression.

Fibro Fog

"For me," says 32-year-old Jane, who is a computer programmer, "this fuzziness in my brain is the hardest to deal with. I'll be looking at someone talking to me; I'll be watching their lips move but have no

Hormones and Fibromyalgia

The symptoms of fibromyalgia are more commonly found in females than in males and may be sensitive to the rise and fall of female hormones. In her book *Screaming to Be Heard: Hormonal Connections Women Suspect . . . and Doctors Ignore,* Dr. Elizabeth Vliet cites a study out of the University of Texas Health Science Center that noted the clinical observation that "in women who developed FMS between the ages of 25 and 40, fully 40 to 50 percent of them were menopausal prior to the onset of FMS—either by surgical menopause or a premature natural menopause."[4] Researchers at the University Hospital Department of Neuroscience Psychiatry in Sweden also found a relationship between hormones and FMS. They report that postmenopausal FMS patients had more severe psychological symptoms than premenopausal patients. These postmenopausal FMS women were also worse off physically and psychologically than postmenopausal healthy women.[5]

idea what they're saying. I simply can't make my brain hold on to their words. It's a terrible thing to just zone out like that and have no control over what registers and what doesn't."

Fibro fog is the term used by many people with fibromyalgia to describe their mental state. Some days their thinking processes are quick and sharp, but other days they just can't focus. The two areas that cause the most problems are short-term memory and attention problems. If you're in a fibro fog, you may lose your keys, forget to turn off the stove, or get in your car and then forget where you're going. Everyone experiences a little of this in day-to-day life, but for people with fibromyalgia it is often a way of life. Fibromyalgics in this state may also have trouble focusing on a subject or a conversation.

Sometimes they may have trouble finding a word or have difficulty performing complex tasks that require intensive attention.

Irritable Bowel Syndrome

"I have a lot of digestive problems along with my fibromyalgia," admits 45-year-old Kurt, a high school teacher, "but the worst is when diarrhea strikes. I can't go anywhere that's more than 10 feet from a bathroom. I just can't control it, and that drives me crazy."

> *Fibro fog is the term used by many people with fibromyalgia to describe their mental state.*

Irritable bowel syndrome (IBS) is common in people with fibromyalgia. A study out of the Harborview Medical Center in Seattle, Washington, asked 22 people with clinically diagnosed fibromyalgia to complete a 138-symptom checklist. The results showed that 77 percent of the study participants had irritable bowel syndrome.[6] The most common symptom of IBS is crampy diarrhea that is often confused with colitis or Crohn's disease. But IBS can also cause constipation, abdominal pain, abdominal gas, and nausea.

Depression

"Sometimes I feel like I just can't hold on anymore," says 40-year-old Maria, a retail clerk. "The pain, the fatigue, and all the other physical problems are too much to bear every day. I feel like I've fallen into a hole and I can't get out."

Because nearly one-third of people with fibromyalgia has a history of depression before being diagnosed with fibromyalgia, medical professionals used to believe that depression was the cause of this condition.[7] Today the American College of Rheumatology has standard diagnostic criteria that confirm FMS as a true illness and not merely psychological in nature.[8] Most people have fibromyalgia for years before their diagnosis and develop depression in response to the chronic pain and fatigue, the lack of medical support, the implication that this condition is "all in their head," and the absence of hope for a normal life. Studies have shown that people with fibromyalgia are no more depressed than those with other chronic, painful, and debilitating disorders, such as rheumatoid arthritis.[9]

There's no doubt that people with fibromyalgia live with circumstances that can trigger depression, but in his 1994 study of fibromyalgia syndrome, Dr. Muhammad Yunus states definitively, "It is clear that abnormal psychological status is not a requirement for development of fibromyalgia."[10] (See chapter 5 for more information on the mind-body relationship in fibromyalgia.)

> *Studies have shown that people with fibromyalgia are no more depressed than those with other chronic, painful, and debilitating disorders, such as rheumatoid arthritis.*

A Long List of Other Symptoms

Many people with fibromyalgia have a variety of other symptoms, problems, and discomforts that seem to be connected to fibromyalgia, but they are not direct symptoms of this syndrome because some people have them and others don't. The list includes the following:

allergies
anxiety
bladder spasms
blurred vision
carpal tunnel
    syndrome
chemical sensitivities
cognitive impairment
coldness of the extremities
crampy abdominal or pelvic pain
depression
dizziness
dry eyes and mouth

feeling of swollen extremities
fingernail ridges
fluid retention
frequent changes in eyeglass
    prescriptions
gastrointestinal disturbances
headaches
hives
impaired coordination
intermittent hearing problems
irritable bladder
joint swelling
memory impairment

mental confusion

migraines

mood swings

muscle tremors

muscle twitching

numbness of the extremities

painful menstruation

palpitations

poor circulation to hands and
feet

poor concentration

premenstrual syndrome

rashes

restless legs syndrome

sensitivity to hot and cold, bright
lights, sounds, smells, cigarette
smoke, perfumes, and especially the weather

skin discoloration

skin tender to the touch

temporomandibular joint
disorder (TMJ)

tingling, itching

urinary urgency or burning

yeast infections

FROM STRONG AND HEALTHY
TO ROCK BOTTOM

Chiropractic physician Dr. Caron Pedersen was diagnosed with fibromyalgia 4 years ago at the age of 31. The year before this diagnosis,
when her symptoms first began, was an emotionally and physically
painful time that changed her personal and professional life forever.

Caron had her own successful practice as a chiropractor and was in
good physical shape. She was very careful about her diet and had always been a strong athlete (she had been a college basketball player).
Caron was an educated person who understood a lot about physical
health and well-being, but she was about to confront something that
would take away her good health and intellect without explanation.

"As an athlete, I knew what getting normally sore was all about,
but I started getting *really* sore. I first noticed that when I went to the
gym to work out, I couldn't do anything without getting stiff and achy,
especially the next day. The pain began on the right side in the rib
cage, and when I went to the doctor she gave me an anti-inflammatory
medication and told me that I had an inflammation of the cartilage in

Fibromyalgia Survey

In an attempt to identify the "typical" person with fibro-myalgia, Ginger H. Ferguson of Forrest General Hospital in Hattiesburg, Mississippi, conducted a survey in 1997 in the tristate area surrounding Tennessee. Of the 280 people with fibromyalgia who were surveyed, the graph below indicates the percentage of those who reported the presence of the following symptoms:

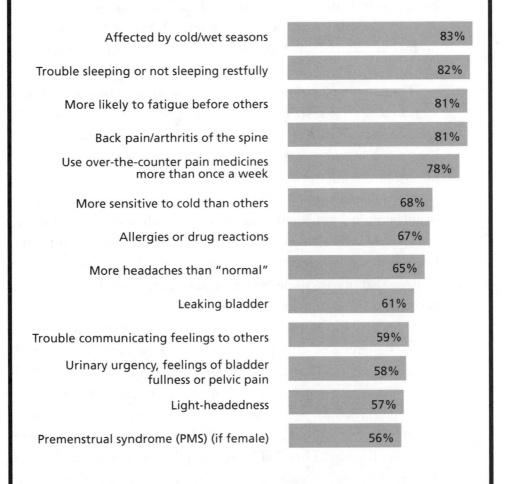

Symptom	Percentage
Affected by cold/wet seasons	83%
Trouble sleeping or not sleeping restfully	82%
More likely to fatigue before others	81%
Back pain/arthritis of the spine	81%
Use over-the-counter pain medicines more than once a week	78%
More sensitive to cold than others	68%
Allergies or drug reactions	67%
More headaches than "normal"	65%
Leaking bladder	61%
Trouble communicating feelings to others	59%
Urinary urgency, feelings of bladder fullness or pelvic pain	58%
Light-headedness	57%
Premenstrual syndrome (PMS) (if female)	56%

Used with permission of Ginger H. Ferguson and Claiborne H. Ferguson between the ribs. But the medication didn't help; in fact, the pain spread to my low back and my legs, and, oddly enough, my face always hurt (and I knew it wasn't because I was smiling too much).

"Soon I got tired of feeling so sore and tired all the time, so I stopped going to the gym and started going to more doctors. But the doctors just blew me off as if I were crazy. They couldn't tell me that I wasn't eating right, or that I didn't get enough exercise, or that I was too stressed, so they'd just say, 'You're just doing too much and making yourself sore and tired.' I couldn't figure out what was going on, but when so many so-called educated medical professionals told me there was nothing really wrong with me, I began to think that I was overreacting, and I tried to ignore what was happening to my body and focused instead on working and getting through each day."

Thinking that maybe her problems were all emotional, Caron went to a psychologist. This mental health professional diagnosed depression, gave Caron prescriptions for medication, and advised her to keep working and to keep her mind off her pain—ignore it. But still the symptoms got worse.

"I would drag myself into work, but then I'd have to cancel my patients because I just couldn't function. My body was so full of pain, I had trouble keeping my balance, and I was getting to the point where I couldn't even remember my patients' names." At the point when she realized that it wasn't safe for her to keep practicing, Caron sold her business—still without knowing what was happening to her.

Soon after she stopped working, Caron tested positive for Epstein-Barr—the virus that causes mononucleosis. Figuring she had a really bad case of mono, Caron gave herself three months to heal her body and get back into shape. Feeling depressed and sick, Caron decided to move to Mexico for a change of scenery. Unfortunately, she had to make this move without the support of her significant other, her family, or her friends. "They said I was crazy; they said I just couldn't handle being in the workplace; they acted like I was wimping out and being very frivolous. There was absolutely nobody to turn to. But I had to do something. There was so much pain all over my body, I thought for sure I was going to die—even if I had to kill myself to do it. Everything I had worked for was gone, so it didn't much matter to me what other people thought of my plans. I figured if I was going to die, I might as well die in a beautiful place."

By this time Caron knew she had something more than Epstein-Barr. "I couldn't sleep at all. I was in indescribable pain; I had headaches and sore throats. Being out in the sun made me feel worse, and I didn't have enough energy to walk around the block. At one point the pain in my leg was so bad I couldn't stand it, so I went to the hospital emergency room where they did all these tests that cost me a whole lot of money, and they found nothing. I had to find out what the hell was going on."

So Caron began her own research into chronic pain and fatigue—which led her to explore chronic fatigue syndrome and fibromyalgia. The most exciting information that came out of this research was that she was not alone. "I began to realize that this was something a lot of people have. I found books and Web sites and medical research that said I was not crazy and that I had an identifiable illness." This information was what Caron needed to decide that she would not go under. "Knowing what I had gave me what I needed to fight back."

> *The most exciting information that came out of Caron's research was that she was not alone.*

Caron's story is typical of the journey so many people with fibromyalgia take as they struggle to find out "what the hell is wrong with me."

A BRIEF HISTORY OF FIBROMYALGIA

You may have been told that you have a "new" disease that medical experts know little about. This is not quite true. Aches and pains in the muscles and joints have been described in documents from biblical times and as muscular rheumatism in the European literature since the 17th century. Since the 1800s, physicians have recognized and written about a condition involving disturbed sleep, fatigue, stiffness, aches, and pains for which there is little or no diagnostic explanation, calling it *muscular rheumatism*. In 1824, a doctor in Edinburgh described tender points. An American psychiatrist wrote in 1880 about a syndrome consisting of general fatigue, widespread pain, and psychological disturbance, calling it *neurasthenia*.[11] Many of these cases (and probably many more since the beginning of humankind) were likely cases of fibromyalgia without the name we now use attached.

In the 20th century, the medical community turned its attention toward naming and defining this condition of diffuse body pain and fatigue. In 1904, Dr. Gowers used the word *fibrositis* to describe the sore spots found in patients with muscular rheumatism. (The Latin root *fibro* means "supportive tissue," and *itis* means "inflammation.") In 1913, the published notes of a lecture on fibrositis given by A. J. Luff pointed out that the symptoms of fibrositis sometimes grew worse in bad weather with lower barometric pressure. He found that extreme changes in temperature, as well as local injuries, fevers, and flu-type infections also increased the severity and frequency of symptoms (many people with fibromyalgia today find the same thing).[12] When it was found in 1947 that there was no evidence of inflammation involved in these patients with widespread pain and localized sore spots, the concept of "psychogenic rheumatism" was proposed in the *Annals of Rheumatoid Disorders*.[13] (It is this decades-old belief that the symptoms of fibromyalgia are all in your head that some physicians still hold fast to today!)

> *A*ches and pains in the muscles and joints have been described in documents from biblical times and as muscular rheumatism in the European literature since the 17th century.

Later, in the 1960s, the word *fibrositis* was used to describe a well-defined syndrome with generalized musculoskeletal aching, tender points at multiple sites, poor sleep, and fatigue (sound familiar?). In

1975, an article was published in *Psychosomatic Medicine* about the musculoskeletal symptoms and sleep disturbance problems in people with fibrositis syndrome.[14]

But the concept of fibromyalgia remained in doubt until 1981, when the first controlled study of the clinical characteristics of this syndrome was performed by Muhammad Yunus, M.D., and his colleagues and published in the journal *Seminars in Arthritis and Rheumatism*.[15] This study showed that multiple symptoms as well as tender points were significantly more common in fibromyalgia than in an age-, sex-, and race-matched normal control group, thus raising fibromyalgia to a recognizable *syndrome* level. A study published in 1987 in the *Journal of the American Medical Association* (*JAMA*) by Don L. Goldenberg, M.D., followed this landmark study that reported on the symptoms, laboratory findings, and treatment results of 118 people with fibromyalgia.[16] (This issue of *JAMA* also set the record straight on correct use of the word *fibromyalgia* rather than *fibrositis*.)

> *The concept of fibromyalgia remained in doubt until 1981, when the first controlled study of the clinical characteristics of this syndrome was performed.*

This promising research, however, was not the end of the confusion. In an article in the *Journal of the American Chiropractic Association*, chiropractor Urscia Mahring describes the typical course of medical "treatment" given to most people with fibromyalgia during the 1980s. She says:

> Fibromyalgia is not a widely supported diagnosis, as medical doctors are not in agreement about its existence even now. In the mid-80s, when I began seeing patients as a student doctor, people would come to us after going to several other doctors who could not find anything wrong with them. Because these patients had a history of having seen multiple doctors, with multiple complaints involving more than one system (musculoskeletal, digestive, perhaps endocrine or immune, and psychological), and because they had shifting areas and intensities of complaints with no apparent causative factors, and

What's in a Name?

Fibromyalgia comes from the Latin: *fibro* meaning "supportive tissue," *myo* for "muscle," and *algia* for "pain." Fibromyalgia is also sometimes called *fibrositis,* a termed coined in 1904 when it was thought that the pain in muscles and surrounding connective tissues was caused by inflammation. However, we now know that inflammation is not a cause of the widespread pain of fibromyalgia, yet you may still see the term used in some literature.

Some researchers in the early 1990s tried to rename the condition *fibromalasia* (meaning discomfort in the soft tissues), but the term did not catch on. Keep it in mind, however, if this word comes up in your research.

Psychogenic rheumatism is a term you should know and be wary of. It is a diagnosis given when a physician believes a patient's widespread pain is due to a psychiatric problem. Although a subgroup of people (about 25 to 35 percent) has a significant psychological prob-

because they tended to appear to be depressed if not downright despondent, and because diagnosis was so extremely frustrating and treatment was like trying to catch the tail of a newt, the sad truth is that people with fibromyalgia easily could be labeled as "symptom magnifiers" and their suffering could be—and often was—discounted and disregarded.

At that time, we diagnosed these patients with fibromyositis or myofibrositis, thinking they had an inflammatory muscle condition. Eventually, though, muscle tissue biopsy revealed a total lack of an inflammatory process. We were also diagnosing these patients as suffering from chronic fatigue syndrome since the symptoms were quite similar.[17]

It has been a long and frustrating search for answers. Finally, in 1990, the American College of Rheumatology classified fibromyalgia lem, fibromyalgia itself is a recognizable collection of symptoms and signs with a physical basis.

Commonly, you will see this condition referred to as *fibromyalgia syndrome* or *FMS* or *FM*. The word *syndrome* is used to describe an illness that consists of a group of symptoms or problems without a known cause. *Fibromyalgia, FMS,* and *FM* are used interchangeably to describe the same illness.

Fibromyalgia has also been called:

- The Invisible Illness (because it is so hard to diagnose)

- Tender Lady Syndrome (a dismissive term used by predominantly male doctors to describe a predominantly female condition)

- Syndrome of the Nineties

- The Irritable Everything Syndrome

as a recognizable syndrome. It defined the term and set standards for diagnosis. Now, for the first time, those with the body aches, fatigue, pain, and misery of this syndrome had the recognition of the medical community.

THE CAUSE

Having a name and a medical classification has given fibromyalgia some long-overdue respect. But it has not answered the most elusive question of all: What causes this condition? There have been many false starts, disappointments, and wrong turns in the search for an explanation, but the good news is that even missteps bring us one day closer to finding out what causes fibromyalgia. The answer to this medical riddle is vital to finding the ultimate cure.

The Role of Genetics

Researchers have found that fibromyalgia seems to run in some families, leading them to speculate that there may be an underlying genetic vulnerability. Some believe that it is common for several generations of a family or many family members of one family to have FMS. A study conducted in the year 2000 with individuals diagnosed with FMS who attended support group meetings throughout Illinois found that 54 of the 145 people (37 percent) in the study reported having relatives with symptoms or a diagnosis of fibromyalgia. Half of this group identified their mothers, and over one-fourth identified their sisters.[18]

> Researchers have found that fibromyalgia seems to run in some families, leading them to speculate that there may be an underlying genetic vulnerability.

Possible Triggers

Whether or not there is a family connection, many people with fibromyalgia can point to a specific event or illness as the "cause" of their condition. There's no doubt that certain events can trigger the symptoms of fibromyalgia. Things such as motor vehicle accidents, periods of prolonged stress, emotional trauma, hormonal changes, viruses, surgery, and certain drugs appear to be capable of flipping the fibro switch in genetically vulnerable people. But many researchers believe that these things are not responsible for the active symptoms.

"I would say that there is little support for many of the 'causes' that have been proposed for fibromyalgia," cautions Dr. Daniel Clauw, chief of the Division of Rheumatology, Immunology, and Allergy at Georgetown University Medical Center and one of the country's leading experts on fibromyalgia. "With time, immune, viral, and other 'causes' of FMS have been overtly disproven, or the tremendous amount of collected data has moved us away from the belief that there is any single environmental exposure (whether an infection, an accident, or an emotional event) that causes fibromyalgia. Most of us now believe that there is some type of dysregulation or sensitization in the way the central nervous system (CNS) operates. I wouldn't say that we have entirely disproven all the alternative causes, but we've certainly moved far away from those toward the more unifying notion that there are several 'triggers' that flip a switch in the central nervous system, causing the various symptoms of fibromyalgia."

Sleep disturbances, for example, are a good example of the way symptoms can be mixed up with possible causes. One hundred percent of people with fibromyalgia in a specific study conducted by J. Rodgers and S. Maurizio reported a sleep disturbance. In this group, nearly three-fourths reported a sleep disturbance every night, with a severity level of 3.7 (with 4.0 being debilitating). Severity of the sleep disorder increased as the number of nights it occurred increased. And it was not surprising that the level of fatigue increased as the level of sleep disturbances increased.[19]

No doubt there is a definite link between FMS and sleep disturbances, but the sleep problems may be a cause and then increase as a symptom, causing a spiral with the disease getting worse. Several studies have shown that if people are deprived of sleep, some of the individuals will develop the symptoms of fibromyalgia. This finding has led some to conclude that sleep dysfunction is the cause of fibromyalgia. However, Dr. Clauw points out that "the data in the sleep literature suggest that a minority of fibromyalgia patients has any significant sleep abnormality, so this probably isn't the place to focus research into the cause of this condition. It seems to me that sleep disturbances are no different than the problems with memory or depression that people with fibromyalgia are known to have; they are all symptoms of fibromyalgia—not the cause."

Other events have been suggested as the "cause" of fibromyalgia but are, at best, triggers. These include the following:

- Viruses (especially the flu and the Epstein-Barr virus)
- Certain types of fungi (such as *Candida albicans*)

- Immune system disorders
- Allergies
- Unrelieved stress
- Nutritional deficiencies
- Heavy metal and chemical toxicity
- Chronic mercury poisoning from amalgam dental fillings
- Muscles especially vulnerable to decreased circulation and minor injury
- Anemia
- Parasites
- Hypoglycemia
- Hypothyroidism

No one has to convince 23-year-old Joanne that there is a relationship among genetics, traumatic events, and her fibromyalgia—her case appears to be a textbook example. Joanne had suffered the pain and fatigue of fibromyalgia for 10 years, but it wasn't until after an automobile accident that the symptoms of fibromyalgia flared with full force and she was finally diagnosed. Then 2 weeks after Joanne was told she had fibromyalgia, Joanne's mother went to a rheumatologist for her arthritis. After talking a while about her health history, which had included pneumonia, lupus, sleep problems, fatigue, and the arthritis, her doctor told her he believed she had fibromyalgia. "We couldn't believe it," remembers Joanne. "Both of us were diagnosed independently of each other!"

History Lessons

The facts about genes and triggers help explain how fibromyalgia develops, but they still don't answer the question, "What causes fibromyalgia?" What is it that keeps these symptoms going for years and

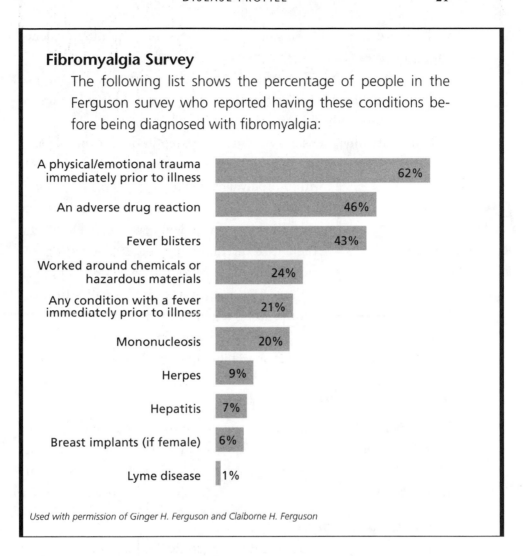

Fibromyalgia Survey

The following list shows the percentage of people in the Ferguson survey who reported having these conditions before being diagnosed with fibromyalgia:

A physical/emotional trauma immediately prior to illness — 62%

An adverse drug reaction — 46%

Fever blisters — 43%

Worked around chemicals or hazardous materials — 24%

Any condition with a fever immediately prior to illness — 21%

Mononucleosis — 20%

Herpes — 9%

Hepatitis — 7%

Breast implants (if female) — 6%

Lyme disease — 1%

Used with permission of Ginger H. Ferguson and Claiborne H. Ferguson

years, long after a genetic switch has been flipped or the initial illness or traumatic event has passed?

If you've done some research looking for the cause, you know there are plenty of possibilities to choose from. Researchers in this field tell us, however, that it's best not to grab onto one single theory or another right now. If you look at the research over the last 10 years, you'll see that at least five or six specific findings have claimed to be the cause of fibromyalgia. Although some scientific evidence supported these cases, further study refuted each one.

Dr. Clauw remembers that 3 years ago everybody with fibromyalgia wanted the tilt-table test after one study found that 95 percent of participants with fibromyalgia tested positive on this test for neurally mediated hypotension. But further testing in other centers found that only a relatively small percentage of people with fibromyalgia really tested positive, and it certainly was not the definitive cause everyone had hoped for. "Every few years," says Dr. Clauw, "there are preliminary studies suggesting we know the cause of fibromyalgia, and with time all of these have been disproven." It takes time for theories to be tested properly and applied to the fibromyalgia population. But still, every once in a while, a new theory will get enough media attention to fill us once again with high hopes.

> *Researchers in this field tell us that it's best not to grab onto one single theory or another right now.*

Today's Headlines

Two very hot theories about the cause of fibromyalgia are making the rounds today: (1) spinal cord compression and (2) mycoplasm bacterium. Both have promising possibilities, but both need much further exploration.

Spinal Cord Compression

In March 2000, the ABC News show *20/20 Friday* threw out what seemed to be a lifeline to the millions of people in America suffering with fibromyalgia. It told of cutting-edge treatment for fibromyalgia that was being practiced by neurosurgeons Dr. Michael Rosner of the University of Alabama in Birmingham and Dr. Dan S. Heffez of the Chicago Institute of Neurosurgery and Neuroresearch. These physicians found that some people with fibromyalgia have the same problem as those with Chiari syndrome and cervical spinal stenosis—a narrowing of the opening at the base of the skull or in the neck that compresses the lower part of the brain or spinal cord. By surgically widening this area, all symptoms significantly improved.

Both doctors became fascinated by the possibility that at least some people who had been diagnosed with chronic fatigue or fibromyalgia indeed had the classic neurosurgical problems that neurosurgeons had been operating on for decades. Eventually Dr. Rosner (who now works out of Park Ridge Hospital in Hendersonville, North Carolina) joined forces with Dr. Heffez, and they now examine and treat patients with the diagnosis of chronic fatigue or fibromyalgia.[20]

During an online chat following the *20/20 Friday* show, Dr. Heffez pointed out a few facts:

- This narrowing in the base of the neck is believed to be a congenital condition that causes the problematic symptoms of fibromyalgia when provoked by trauma or accident. Seventy percent of treated patients reported a history of trauma.

- This is not a cure but a method of improving the quality of life by lessening symptoms.

- The less time someone has experienced the symptoms of fibromyalgia, the more successful the results.

- Eighty-eight percent of the surgeries resulted in meaningful improvement to the patient.[21]

However, before you run to a neurologist asking for a diagnostic MRI (magnetic resonance imaging), you should know that this theory recently took a backward step when the results of a pilot spinal cord compression surveillance study sponsored by the National Fibromyalgia Research Association were reported at the American College of Rheumatology (ACR) annual meeting in the fall of 2000. Dr. Clauw took part in this study and finds the results disappointing. "Our study found that there wasn't any higher rate of Chiari malformations or cervical stenosis in fibromyalgia patients than in the general population. In fact, there were more people with these structural abnormalities of the spine who had no symptoms at all than those who had fibromyalgia.

"This is only a single study," he adds, "so I'm not in any way saying this theory should be discarded, but even the biggest proponents of this theory are suggesting that only individuals with an abnormal neurological exam should be given a diagnostic MRI. In fact, many of the patient advocacy groups who were originally very excited about this finding are recommending against patients having MRIs routinely."

Once again the research into the cause of FMS seems to have taken two steps forward and one step back—but even that puts us ahead of where we were before the research began.

Mycoplasm Bacterium

In a study published in the journal *Medical Sentinel*, Dr. Garth L. Nicolson and colleagues present a compelling case arguing that the disorders chronic fatigue syndrome (CFS), fibromyalgia, Gulf War illness (GWI), and a number of other chronic illnesses stem from a similar cause—infection by a primitive bacterium called a *mycoplasm*.[22]

Mycoplasma is a genus of microscopic organisms that lack a rigid cell wall, falling somewhere between a virus and a bacterium. Many are pathogens, causing diseases such as mycoplasma pneumonia, one type of sexually transmitted infection of the urethra called *nongonococcal urethritis*, as well as infections of the heart (endocarditis, myocarditis), and, some researchers speculate, severe asthma. Mycoplasma can exist harmlessly in the mouth and alimentary canal, but, as Nicolson writes, "when they penetrate into the blood and tissues, they may be able to cause or promote a variety of acute or chronic illnesses."

Nicolson's team compared people with CFS, fibromyalgia, GWI, and rheumatoid arthritis to healthy people, looking for signs of mycoplasma in the subjects' white blood cells (leukocytes). In their study of 203 people with fibromyalgia, Nicolson and his colleagues found almost 70 percent of those suffering symptoms were infected with the bacterium (or at least showed signs of mycoplasma DNA), in contrast to 9 percent of the healthy control group of 70 people.

In his online article, Dr. Mark Young, associate chair of Physical Medicine and Rehabilitation at the Maryland Rehabilitation Center and a member of the faculty of the Sinai/Johns Hopkins Physical Medicine and Rehabilitation training program, expresses guarded optimism about the new study: "The bacteria could be present as a cofactor, and not the cause of the many symptoms patients experience."[23] Most researchers agree that it is still unclear whether mycoplasma infection is the cause of these chronic illnesses, a cofactor, or merely an opportunistic infection resulting from exposure and the patient's already weakened immune system.

Dr. Clauw believes that when all is said and done, we may find that the Chiari syndrome, cervical stenosis, and mycoplasma infections may be responsible for symptoms in a small percentage of people with fibromyalgia, but by no means will they be the definitive cause of fibromyalgia. There is still much work to be done.

> *It is still unclear whether mycoplasma infection is the cause of chronic illnesses, a cofactor, or merely an opportunistic infection resulting from exposure and the patient's already weakened immune system.*

New Directions

Over the years a long list of possible causes of fibromyalgia has been studied and proposed—none with definitive results. Now, finally, there is reason for hope. Dr. Clauw tells us, "We're learning things more rapidly than we ever have before. There is near unanimity within the scientific community that fibromyalgia is some type of disturbance in the function of the central nervous system. There was a lot of money that was poured into looking for viral or immune abnormalities that were felt to be responsible for the illness. But now those studies are largely being abandoned, at least at the federal level." This conclusion is a major breakthrough that has changed the party line, which thought that fibro was probably caused by infections or immune system disorders. It allows researchers to focus in one area, making it more likely that a definitive cause can be found.

But don't begin celebrating just yet. Finding the exact disturbance in the central nervous system that causes fibromyalgia is not an easy task. The central nervous system consists of the brain and spinal cord and is composed of a vast system of receptors and fibers that receives and sends signals to all parts of the body. The CNS is connected to a peripheral nervous system which connects nerves to most of our tissues, especially to muscle, bone and joints. Many things can go wrong within this system. Research into the role of the nervous system in fibromyalgia is focusing on many possible problems. The two most promising possibilities are altered pain perception and malfunction in two key CNS systems.

Altered Pain Perception

Jon Russell, M.D., Ph.D., of the University of Texas Health Sciences Center in San Antonio, suspects that the persistent pain of fibromyalgia leads to a heightened sensitivity to pain that spreads far beyond the site of the original injury. In her article "I Hurt All Over" in *Psychology Today*, Mirinda Kossoff reports that Dr. Russell says, "In fibromyalgia we don't see discernible tissue damage that would cause pain. It appears that within the central nervous system, something has happened to the pain perception process."[24] In studies of people with FMS, Russell and his colleagues have detected abnormal levels of several chemicals that relay signals around the nervous system. The most dramatic, says Russell, is an elevated level of the neurotransmitter substance P, which the body normally releases into the spinal cord when it is injured. Abnormally high levels of substance P cause neurons to send pain messages to the brain, even when there is no pain-causing injury in any part of the body. In addition, concentrations of three other brain chemicals—dopamine, norepinephrine, and serotonin—that are necessary to regulate levels of substance P appear to be abnormally low in people with FMS.

The abnormal level of serotonin could itself be a cause of fibromyalgia. Serotonin is a neurotransmitter in the brain associated with a calming, anxiety-reducing action. Lower levels of serotonin cause a lower pain threshold. Depressed levels of serotonin may also help explain why FMS is more prevalent in women than men. For as yet unexplained reasons, women naturally appear to produce less serotonin than men, notes Russell, which might account for the generally lower pain threshold in women.

Russell, like other scientists working in the field, predicts that fibromyalgia will follow the path of other mysterious ailments. Twenty years ago, he notes, rheumatoid arthritis was considered a psychological illness, its symptoms exacerbated by stress and life changes. Today, we know that stress has nothing to do with it. "Fibromyalgia is undergoing the same transition," says Russell.[25]

> *Concentrations of three other brain chemicals—dopamine, norepinephrine, and serotonin—that are necessary to regulate levels of substance P appear to be abnormally low in people with FMS.*

Malfunction in Two Key CNS Systems

According to some studies, people with fibromyalgia may have malfunctions in two key systems of the central nervous system:

1. The autonomic nervous system (the automatic or self-controlling mechanism)

2. The HPA axis (which regulates production of certain hormones and the body's response to stress)

Boston researcher Gail K. Adler, M.D., Ph.D., and fellow Harvard Medical School researchers discovered that in some women with FMS, the complex brain-to-body pathway involving the hypothalamus, the pituitary, and the adrenal glands (the HPA axis) is damaged. As a result, it does not properly regulate production of cortisol, a hormone with widespread effects throughout the body. Some participants had decreased function of the HPA axis, while others had an excess of activity. In both cases, the levels of key hormones were affected, resulting in the symptoms of fibromyalgia.[26]

The Air We Breathe

In a 1999 article in the *Journal of Environmental Health,* Emily Wilson reported an unusual cluster of fibromyalgia cases among the faculty at an educational facility in Florida. These faculty members were from the dental, nursing, and allied health sciences disciplines, and all worked in the same building. When it was noticed anecdotally that 10 faculty members had been diagnosed with fibromyalgia and reports from professional consulting engineers indicated that ventilation of the building was inadequate for the laboratory activities that were conducted in the building, the local health department director sent a request for assistance to the bureau chief of environmental epidemiology at the Florida State Department of Health. The results of their study found that an exceptionally high 13

In support of this finding, the National Institute of Arthritis and Musculoskeletal and Skin Diseases (NIAMS) is funding a study testing the belief that abnormally low levels of cortisol may be associated with fibromyalgia. These researchers believe that people whose bodies make inadequate amounts of cortisol experience many of the same symptoms as people with fibromyalgia.[27]

In this research, the pieces seem to fit. The HPA axis and the autonomic nervous system are the major pathways for body responses to stressful conditions that are known to trigger fibromyalgia—trauma and infection, for example. Both systems are influenced by genetic and environmental factors and by chronic illness. And both systems affect pain, alertness, gastrointestinal motility, and fatigue. It is logical that if something goes wrong in these systems, the results can be one or all of the many symptoms of fibromyalgia.

Many studies are underway, and many theories are yet to be proven, but in the end, Dr. Clauw believes this: "I think we will find that the cause of fibromyalgia is a dysfunction in these various areas of percent of the faculty in the "sick" building had fibromyalgia. Because this rate is certainly higher than the expected 2 percent of the general population who have fibromyalgia, the results seem to indicate that fibromyalgia may be caused by an environmental toxin in the air we breathe.

However, this one situation has not caused much interest in the medical research community for two reasons: No other study has found any relationship between air quality and the incidence of fibromyalgia, and the 13 percent occurrence rate may not be exceptional when all facts are considered. Eighty-five percent of the study respondents were females, and females are seven times more likely than males to have fibromyalgia. Simple math indicates that the 13 percent occurrence may not be exceptional after all.[20]

the central nervous system. A lot of the disorders that are accompanied by this type of dysfunction—whether it's dyslexia, migraines, or irritable bowel syndrome—cause symptoms but don't have a structural basis for their occurrence. It is likely that something is wrong with functions of various components of the central nervous system that leads to the symptoms we see. I don't think it's going to be a single cause for all people with fibromyalgia. I believe we will find that there are many ways people end up in the same clinical state." Hence, FMS may be a multifactorial illness, with many causes. This has been the lesson with other illnesses such as cancer.

WHO GETS FIBROMYALGIA?

If you believe you have fibromyalgia, not only are you not crazy—you are not alone. The American College of Rheumatology tells us that fibromyalgia may affect about 2 percent of the U.S. population—that's three to six million people. It occurs seven times more frequently in women than in men. Some experts estimate that approximately 8 percent of women have fibromyalgia. It is the second most common diagnosis in rheumatology clinics, behind osteoarthritis.

Although fibromyalgia is found in children (see details later in this chapter) and the elderly, it is most frequently diagnosed between the ages of 40 and 50. That means if you are a middle-aged female, you are smack in the target group of people who are likely to get fibromyalgia.

Just the Facts

According to the American College of Rheumatology, the percentage of the American population who have fibromyalgia is:

2.0% overall

3.4% of women

0.5% of men

Race

It's difficult to say whether one race is more prone to this medical condition than others. Most people with fibromyalgia described in the literature are white, but it should not be assumed that this is a disease of Caucasian people only. It is more likely that the studies on white people are the result of clinic and referral biases. There is a study of fibromyalgia in the Japanese population and another in the South African black population, so it would seem that this syndrome knows no race or global boundary.[29]

Fibromyalgia in Children

A form of fibromyalgia called *juvenile primary fibromyalgia syndrome* (JPFS) is increasingly appearing in children and adolescents. Dr. Yukiko Kimura, chief of pediatric rheumatology at Hackensack University Medical Center in New Jersey, has studied JPFS and believes that it is a relatively common cause of pain and disability in children. Yet he believes that JPFS often escapes timely detection or is not noticed at all.[30]

Although data regarding the incidence of musculoskeletal pain in normal children are scarce, the facts indicate that JPFS is not a "rare" pediatric condition:

- At one pediatric rheumatology center, Drs. Yunus and Masi found that JPFS was diagnosed almost as frequently as juvenile rheumatoid arthritis.[31] One study looked at 548 children from three public schools in Mexico. A total of 24 (4.4 percent) complained of some form of musculoskeletal pain. JFPS was diagnosed in 7 of those 24 children.[32]

- Drs. Bowyer and Roettcher found that 5.1 percent of all children with rheumatic disease in 25 pediatric rheumatology centers in the United States had fibromyalgia.[33]

Remember Joanne, whose mother also has fibromyalgia? She is one of the people who knows from experience that children get fibromyalgia. In 1999, at age 23, Joanne was diagnosed with fibromyalgia, but she knows that she has had the symptoms of this condition since she was a child. After having frequent bouts of the flu with fevers of 103 degrees, she began to suffer digestive problems and chronic constipation. As a young teen, she lived on stool softeners, laxatives, and enemas. She laughs now as she remembers, "You can imagine how upset I was about getting enemas from my mother when I was 13!" Soon afterward, Joanne noticed that she felt very tired all the time, and her knees often hurt. "I was out of school for a two-week period, sleeping 16 hours a day. I just didn't have the strength to lift my body out of bed. When I would finally go back to school with the explanation that 'I was too tired to come to school,' I didn't get any sympathy for my condition or leniency for the work that was due. Even my sisters resented me for staying home to lie around and do nothing. My teenage years were totally controlled by this problem. Eventually I withdrew from my friends, and I became distant and quiet—I felt alone and kind of hopeless."

During those years, neither Joanne nor her doctor had a clue about what was causing her to feel so miserable. "My doctor told me to do exercises to strengthen my knees so they wouldn't hurt so much, and he tested me for mononucleosis five different times—always with negative results. He would just pat me on the shoulder and say something like, 'I guess you're just tired.'"

But it was soon more than just fatigue and sore knees. Joanne started having frequent headaches and not only her knees but also her hips and neck area began to ache. Then by the time she entered college, Joanne found she was fighting brain fog. "I just couldn't concentrate at all to study or to pay attention in the classroom. Thinking maybe I had attention deficit disorder, I went to the psychologist on campus for some help. She didn't feel I had an attention disorder and just encouraged me to keep trying to study hard. I went to my college mentor and explained my concerns about working so hard and yet not getting anywhere in my studies; he, too, told me to just keep at it."

> *Most children are 11 to 13 years old at the time JPFS is diagnosed but have had symptoms for months or years beforehand.*

Despite these assurances that nothing was wrong with her, Joanne began to suspect that something was very wrong when she noticed that her symptoms ran in cycles. She would go through periods each year when the fatigue and body aches and brain fog were overwhelming and then other periods when she would feel almost fine. Then something happened to trigger a major bout: Joanne was in a car accident.

After her car was hit from behind and pushed into the car in front of her, the list of physical complaints grew. "The fatigue returned; my whole body ached; my neck hurt terribly; I developed sleep apnea that kept me from getting a good night's sleep, and I also had TMJ." Joanne's doctor referred her to a physical therapist and a biofeedback specialist for her pain, but they all assumed her symptoms were caused by the car accident. "I can't help but feel a little angry," Joanne now admits. "If only I had been properly diagnosed when I was young, I think my whole life would have been different."

Fortunately, today JPFS is slightly better known in the medical community, and more children are getting the proper diagnosis early. Most children are 11 to 13 years old at the time JPFS is diagnosed but have had symptoms for months or years beforehand. Symptoms may begin when the child is just 5 or 6 years old. Of the 33 children diagnosed in one study, 4 (12 percent) were 5 to 6 years old, 5 (15 percent) were 7 to 9 years old, and 4 (12 percent) were 10 to 12 years old. The remaining patients were in their midteens.[34] Many aspects of JPFS are similar to adult-onset fibromyalgia: The symptoms are the same. Girls and young women appear to be affected more often than boys and young men. And there may be a tendency for FMS and JPFS to occur in families. (In a study of 34 children with JPFS, 71 percent of the mothers had previously undiagnosed FMS.[35])

In one important way, however, JPFS appears to be different from adult-onset fibromyalgia. Studies are finding that young persons with JPFS may have better prospects for improvement or remission than adults with FMS. In a 1995 study of 338 healthy schoolchildren, JPFS was diagnosed in 21 of them. These children were monitored but not treated. Of the 15 who were contacted at the 30-month follow-up, only 4 (27 percent) still had evidence of FMS.[36] In another study conducted in 1999, JPFS was diagnosed in 22 of 1,756 healthy students. A year later, only 9 of the 16 untreated children who were contacted for follow-up still had symptoms.[37] Drs. Yunus and Masi have found that the average time to improvement for children is 18.8 months.[38] These findings contrast with studies that have been done in adults, which show a higher rate of persistent symptoms. In two investigations, 60 to 97 percent of adults with FMS still had symptoms at 1 year of follow-up.[39] We do not yet know whether after childhood remission the symptoms of fibromyalgia will return in adulthood, but it does seem that the prognosis is better for children than adults.

> *Studies are finding that young persons with JPFS may have better prospects for improvement or remission than adults with FMS.*

THE EXPECTED COURSE OF FIBROMYALGIA

The course of fibromyalgia is usually unpredictable. Some people start with a few vague aches and pains that progress over the years to full-blown fibromyalgia. Others experience the full, unrestrained force of excruciating pain and debilitating fatigue immediately after a traumatic incident such as a car accident and hold onto those problems long after all other physical injuries have passed. These different experiences make it impossible to say how one person's case will progress.

It is common for fibromyalgia to have cycles of flare-ups and seeming remission. In fact, even some weather conditions may affect symptoms: People usually do worse in cold weather and can sometimes predict rain (because symptoms are worsened by humidity and falling barometric pressure). Sleep disturbances can also affect symptoms: On days following a good night's sleep, the symptoms may be less noticeable, but after a sleepless night will flare. In any event, the symptoms of FMS are likely to be detectable at varying levels of intensity throughout a person's life.

> *The symptoms of FMS are likely to be detectable at varying levels of intensity throughout a person's life.*

Some statistics tell us that one-third of people with fibromyalgia are partially or totally disabled by this illness. "What is most disabling," says Steve Thorson, a Fibromyalgia Network representative, "is that people with fibromyalgia don't know how they're going to feel from day to day. There are times when they can work very competently, but then there are other times when they just can't function at all because they are in a pain flare or fatigued. Their bodies are undependable—and that is very disabling."

The Good Day/Bad Day Roller-Coaster

If you have fibromyalgia, you know you have some good days and some just awful days. On a recent awful day, Mary was sure it couldn't get much worse. "I have been plagued with reflux, heartburn, nausea and vomiting, and diarrhea. I can't sleep for the frequent trips to bathroom. And I have never had gas like this before. The muscles in my arms and legs are spasming most of the day and night. My back hurts horribly and unforgivingly. I have had a headache for a week. The fog is starting to get to me. I write everything down and forget where I wrote it. My feet feel like they are bruised all over and can't stand to be touched. I can't even stand on them. I really wish for one of those good days I used to have."

On those good days Mary's irritable bowel is calm, and because she catches a few hours' sleep, her days are more manageable. "There are some days when I can almost function normally. The pain medication actually works, and I can think clearly. My feet almost always hurt, but on good days I can walk around and get some things done. I can go shopping and make myself a good meal. Although I feel tired, it's not the kind of tired that keeps me down and out in bed. I know this isn't what the rest of the world would call a good day, but for me it's what I live for."

What those with fibromyalgia also live for is competent and empathetic doctors who can diagnosis their condition correctly and put them on the right path to healing. The following chapters will guide you through the diagnostic and treatment process for this syndrome that at this time is considered a chronic, manageable condition—but not curable. A cure is our hope for tomorrow.

CHAPTER 2

Diagnosis

THE PROCESS FOR diagnosing fibromyalgia that used to make people jump through hoops in the past has finally landed in a sane place. Now that many medical professionals clearly understand that fibromyalgia does exist and has identifiable characteristics, you should be able to go to a medical doctor and get a definitive diagnosis. This is a major change from the dragged-out, doctor hopping, "Nobody believes me" process of just a few years ago. Medical researchers like Muhammad B. Yunus, M.D., FACP, FACR, professor of medicine at the University of Illinois College of Medicine (who is credited with popularizing the term *fibromyalgia* through his writings and presentations in the early 1980s), believes "this syndrome can be easily and reliably diagnosed by an experienced practitioner." This is good news.

The bad news is that far too many doctors are not "experienced practitioners"; they still do not know how to recognize the symptoms of fibromyalgia or do not believe that the condition really exists. It's true that fibromyalgia has no structural, identifiable problem. There is no diagnostic test for FMS. Many diagnostic tests—blood, urine, x ray, CAT scan, and magnetic resonance imaging (MRI)—are performed on people with fibromyalgia with no conclusive evidence that there is anything wrong. In fact, many insist that FMS cannot even be called a "disease" because it lacks clinical evidence of any structural or biochemical abnormality. Like tension headaches and irritable bowl syndrome, the exact physiological nature of the problem has not been found, giving it a bad name among some in the medical community. The diagnosis must be made from the patient's history and the combination of symptoms, what doctors call making a "clinical diagnosis."

OVERCOMING A CREDIBILITY PROBLEM

Despite the advances that have been made in the general understanding of what fibromyalgia is and how to diagnose it, its credibility problem has made it very difficult for some people to get an accurate diagnosis in a reasonable amount of time. According to Debra Buchwald, M.D., at the University of Washington, "patients go to many kinds of physicians in their search for help. From the frustrated provider's point of view, they are doctor shopping. From the patient's point of view, they are simply trying to get better." Based on a survey by Dr. Buchwald, undiagnosed FMS patients arriving at her clinic paid an average of 27 visits to a health care provider during the previous year.[1] This can't be good for a condition that is aggravated and even sustained by stress!

> *Now that many medical professionals clearly understand that fibromyalgia does exist and has identifiable characteristics, you should be able to go to a medical doctor and get a definitive diagnosis.*

Some blame the difficulty of getting a correct diagnosis on insurance companies. For someone with a serious, chronic illness such as fibromyalgia, proper diagnosis cannot be made in the average 6 minute office visit typical in managed care programs. And in practices in which the physician is paid a set monthly fee by the insurance carrier for every patient, treating too many time-intensive illnesses can be economic suicide. But Dr. Joseph E. Scherger, dean of the College of Medicine at Florida State University in Tallahassee, and former editor in chief of *Hippocrates* (the primary care journal from the publishers of the

New England Journal of Medicine), isn't so quick to point that finger. "Insurance companies may be part of the problem," he says, "but the reality is that if the doctor defines how he works by what he gets paid, this is already a problem. Some patients are quick and simple; others are long and complicated. The insurance company will pay the same whether it's a short or long visit, but a long visit cuts down on the number of patients the doctor will see in that day and therefore on the day's profits." Because fibromyalgia isn't a "quick and easy" disease, many doctors avoid these patients.

James expected to have trouble getting insurance coverage for his mysterious symptoms because he works for a health insurance company and knows how claims for chronic illnesses are handled, but he didn't foresee the trouble he would have finding a physician who could accurately diagnose his problem.

> *Insurance companies may be part of the problem, but the reality is that if the doctor defines how he works by what he gets paid, this is already a problem.*
>
> —JOSEPH E. SCHERGER, M.D.

At first the 46-year-old thought it was just the aches and pains of aging that were giving him trouble, so it's hard for James to nail down when he first started having the symptoms that made him think something was wrong. "About two years ago my biggest problem was my sore shoulder blades when I woke up in the morning. Then over time, I felt a weakness in my legs. Then one day I sat down on the floor to help my kids wrap Christmas presents, and my leg joints just locked. I had to get on my knees and slowly lift myself. After that I started getting severe pains in my ribs. As soon as I woke up in the morning, I had to get out of bed immediately because I couldn't stand the pain. My elbows, too, hurt so badly that it was hard to wash my face in the morning. But after about 15 minutes of stretching, most of the pain would be gone, so this wasn't debilitating—just extremely annoying. And I was so tired—probably because I was getting only about four hours of sleep a night. Although I was still functioning everyday, I decided to go to my doctor to find out what was going on." At this point James had no idea what he was getting into.

James's general practitioner (GP) checked him out and found nothing wrong, so he referred him to a neurologist. The neurologist checked the nerve function and found that the upper extremities were fine, but the lower ones were weak. "Because at that time I was self-medicating with alcohol, he told me to stop drinking and that should stop the discomfort. So I did. Over a year later the pain was worse."

The GP then sent James to a rheumatologist. He did a general exam and ordered blood work. "I was checked for lupus, hepatitis C, Lyme disease, and God knows what else—about $2,000 worth of blood work in all." In the end the rheumatologist found nothing wrong. In conversation, James brought up the possibility of fibromyalgia. His sister-in-law has suffered for years with this condition, so he was somewhat familiar with what she had been through. He also had some professional dealings with this syndrome and was familiar with the term *fibromyalgia*. "I remember 15 years ago when it was a knockdown, drag-out fight to get an insurance company to pay any benefits for this. Now it takes only about five rounds to get a claim paid, so I guess that's progress." The doctor said he wouldn't rule out fibromyalgia, but because its diagnosis was a process of elimination, it would take time to determine. However, the doctor noticed a swollen gland on James's neck and sent him to an endocrinologist.

> **Just the Facts**
> According to rheumatologists, FMS is one of the most common diagnoses in rheumatology ambulatory practice; however, in general practice it remains one of the most underreported.[2]

The endocrinologist withdrew fluid from the gland for examination. The results were inconclusive, and he advised James to have it checked every six months. But he offered no opinion about what could be causing the swelling and had no idea why James's body was in such pain.

James went back to the neurologist, who reexamined him and said, "There's nothing at all wrong with you." He gave James some antidepressants and sent him home. After six weeks James felt no relief so he called him back. That's when this doctor gave up. "I don't think I'm the one who can help you," he said.

James went back to his GP, who gave him an anti-inflammatory drug—which provided no results. As of this writing he has scheduled an MRI to rule out problems in the brain and central nervous system. "That's where I am now," says James with a shrug. "I honestly don't know what's wrong. Maybe this is more psychosomatic than real and it will just go away. Right now I'm really clueless."

The only thing for sure about James's case is that he is not alone. Thousands like him right now are traveling through this bewildering journey. Maybe he has fibromyalgia; maybe he doesn't. Maybe it's all in his head—most likely it's not. But unfortunately, as is the case with so many people with chronic pain, his journey through the world of "inconclusive results" has already been a long and tiring one.

Getting an accurate diagnosis of fibromyalgia doesn't have to be so difficult. A pamphlet published by the Fibromyalgia Network cites a study that reassures us that a physician trained in diagnosing FMS can do it even under difficult circumstances. The pamphlet says:

> The 1990 multi-center criteria study evaluated a total of 558 patients of which 265 were classified as controls. These control individuals weren't your typical healthy "normals." They were age- and sex-matched patients with neck pain syndrome, low back pain, local tendinitis, trauma-related pain syndromes, rheumatoid arthritis, lupus, osteoarthritis of the knee or hand, and other painful disorders. These patients all had some symptoms that mimic FMS, but the trained examiners were not foiled—they hand-picked the FMS patients out of the "chronically ill" melting pot with an accuracy of 88 percent.[3]

If you suspect you may have fibromyalgia but are having trouble getting an accurate diagnosis, your first move must be to find the right medical professional.

The Doctors' Points-of-View

How do physicians feel about seeing patients with fibromyalgia? Look at what some have to say:

- **Frances Leung, M.D.,** a rheumatologist from Toronto, Canada, who has a special interest in FMS: "Dealing with fibromyalgic patients is a problem for some doctors. Many of my colleagues don't want to deal with FMS patients because they are viewed as demanding and they never seem to get better. It's a topic we doctors feel embarrassed about because we are so impotent."[4]

- **Daniel Clauw, M.D.,** chief of the Division of Rheumatology, Immunology, and Allergy at Georgetown University Medical Center: "It's not totally accepted within the entire medical community. Some physicians like to be able to have objective diagnostic tests to understand an illness and we don't have those for fibromyalgia. Also, some doctors develop opinions about illnesses and physiologic mechanisms early in their training, which are hard to change—even if there are subsequent data suggesting that it's different from what they originally thought."[5]

FINDING THE RIGHT DOCTOR

Finding the right doctor is vitally important to obtaining an accurate diagnosis of fibromyalgia. A needs assessment study reported in *Family and Community Health* confirmed that it is common for individuals to have FMS symptoms for years before the condition is diagnosed. It took many people in this study up to 6 years after onset of their symptoms to receive the diagnosis of FMS. Twenty-eight percent experienced pain for 15 to 50 years before they received a diagnosis![8]

As bleak as this sounds, the new hope for this situation is pointed out by Steve Thorson, a representative of the Fibromyalgia Network.

- **Steven Blum, M.D.,** a primary physician at the Pain Center at Rush North Shore Medical Center in Chicago and an assistant professor in anesthesiology and family medicine at Rush Medical College: "Really the best person to care for FMS patients is one who is interested in them. The exact medical specialty is not important. They can be from any area. Heck, I'm an anesthesiologist!"[6]

- **Joseph E. Scherger, M.D., M.P.H.,** dean of the College of Medicine at Florida State University, Tallahassee: "In general, rheumatologists hate the condition because the lab tests are all normal."

- **Arthur J. Hartz, M.D., Ph.D.,** professor and research director of the Department of Family Medicine at the University of Iowa College of Medicine in Iowa City: "Doctors have more of a medical model for treating strep throat or heart disease or other physical ailments, and they have some medical models for treating psychological problems like depression, but when it comes to unexplained illness or symptoms, they don't really have an approach that is as established."[7]

"Ten years ago, it would easily take eight years and 10 to 20 doctors to get the diagnosis," he says, "but today it shouldn't be difficult to find a doctor who can accurately diagnose fibromyalgia. Now you have organizations like ours who can refer people to doctors, there are more articles out there, and doctors are more familiar with the condition. Even if a doctor doesn't know how to pinpoint fibromyalgia, he or she should be able to refer the patient to someone who can."

Dr. Scherger, who frequently speaks on fibromyalgia, agrees, but he also knows the search for the right doctor is not simple or routine. He believes that people who think they may have fibromyalgia have to take an active part in finding a very comprehensive physician. He suggests that you look for a doctor who:

- Is willing to take the time to really understand you
- Will listen to you
- Has a good understanding of the nature of the condition
- Shows a sense of compassion
- Is a holistic-health-oriented provider willing to take an hour to talk to you on your first visit
- Is willing to take a biological, psychological, social, and even spiritual way of helping you find the pathway to getting better

People who think they may have fibromyalgia have to take an active part in finding a very comprehensive physician.

And he adds that you *don't* want a doctor who immediately pulls out the prescription pad, who wants to do a zillion tests, or who allows only short office visits—these are not doctors who can help someone with FMS.

Megan, a 38-year-old freelance writer and mother of three, found out very quickly that she had to be very proactive and determined to find the right doctor. Megan's journey from acute symptoms to finding the right doctor was "only" 6 months long—but there's no doubt that if she did not have such a strong will and sense of self-confidence, she'd still be out there wondering "what the heck is wrong with me."

In November 1997 at the age of 35, Megan came down with a killer case of the flu—body aches, fever, and general all-around weakness put her in bed for a week. Never one to run to the doctor, Megan waited it out, expecting to recover any day, but then she was hit with what she thought was a urinary tract infection. Finally, she dragged herself to the doctor, who gave her antibiotics and sent her back to bed. After another week, there was no change in the flu or urinary symptoms, so Megan went back to the doctor.

Thinking the infection may have spread to her kidneys, Megan was referred to a urologist. He prescribed a new antibiotic and a pain reliever and dye tests on the kidney. When all reports were put together, the urologist sat down with Megan and said, "There's absolutely nothing wrong with your bladder or kidney." Megan remembers sitting there staring at him in tears. "I know there's something wrong. I've been sick and in pain for four weeks." Well, the doctor sympathized with her distress, but he was sure the problem wasn't in the urinary tract.

At this point, the primary care physician decided to do a series of blood tests to rule out a number of possible causes. She tested Megan for various rheumatoid and muscular diseases such as arthritis, Lyme disease, multiple sclerosis, and lupus. She also tested for hepatitis and liver disease. But nothing came up positive. This wasn't the end of the search for Megan, however; her body was telling her loud and clear that something was definitely wrong, and she was determined to find out what it was.

> **Referral Resource**
>
> You can obtain a list of doctors in your state who treat fibromyalgia patients from:
>
> **Fibromyalgia Network**
> P.O. Box 31750
> Tucson, AZ 85751
> Phone: (800) 853-2929

By this time, Megan had started having pain in her joints and especially bad spinal and back pain. Figuring it might just be leftover flu aches, she tried to ignore it at first, but after a month she was sure something else was going on. Her doctor then sent her for liver tests and a series of other tests ("I don't remember exactly what they were for"). When Megan went to the office to get these results, her doctor's partner met with her. This was a young woman whom Megan had never met before. "She looked at me and said, 'Your blood work is fine. There is nothing wrong with you.' I said, 'I know something is drastically wrong. I have not been able to function for two months.' Then this doctor who had known Megan for just a few minutes recommended physical therapy for her posture, psychotherapy, and an antidepressant. "I couldn't believe I was being dismissed because my blood said nothing was wrong, even though my own words and my experience and my pain were saying that there was."

Completely at a loss for answers, one of Megan's friends wondered aloud whether she might have fibromyalgia—the pattern of symptoms seemed to fit. After some research, Megan found that a clinical diagnosis of fibromyalgia could not be made until the symptoms had become "chronic" so she decided to wait a few more months until she proposed this idea to her doctor. During this time, she tried to relieve her symptoms with various supplements, homeopathic drugs, and chiropractic work, but the symptoms continued to worsen. In fact, now the problems were cognitive as well as physical. Megan remembers. "I just couldn't think clearly and concentrate anymore; I just couldn't get my thoughts together. This was very frightening."

> *This doctor who had known Megan for just a few minutes recommended physical therapy for her posture, psychotherapy, and an antidepressant.*

Finally, after waiting six months, Megan went back to her doctor and asked whether it was possible that she might have fibromyalgia. The answer was abrupt but to the point: "I don't believe in fibromyalgia." But the doctor did concede that it might not be a bad idea to check for rheumatoid disease. Without much hope, Megan made an appointment with a rheumatologist.

"After all those months of suffering and all those doctors and tests," says Megan with amazement, "this doctor listened to my history, gave me the tender point test that's used to diagnose fibromyalgia, and within 10 minutes said, 'You have fibromyalgia.'

"I felt this immediate rush of relief. This word, this label, meant I was not insane and there really was something wrong with me—and it was not cancer or some other fatal disease. It's amazing that I could hear that I have this chronic, incurable disease and yet feel relief after having been told for so long that I was crazy."

Megan's sense of relief is natural after having been told by her primary care doctor that there is no such thing as fibromyalgia. This attitude is quite common. But if this happens to you, Dr. Scherger doesn't think this means you necessarily have to jump ship right away. "It's impossible for one person to be all things to you for your whole life," he says. "Even a good personal physician may not be the right

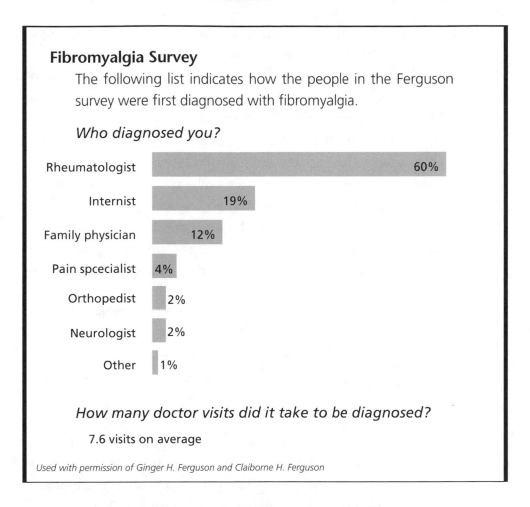

Fibromyalgia Survey

The following list indicates how the people in the Ferguson survey were first diagnosed with fibromyalgia.

Who diagnosed you?

Rheumatologist 60%
Internist 19%
Family physician 12%
Pain spcecialist 4%
Orthopedist 2%
Neurologist 2%
Other 1%

How many doctor visits did it take to be diagnosed?

7.6 visits on average

Used with permission of Ginger H. Ferguson and Claiborne H. Ferguson

person to help you with everything. But if you have trusted this doctor in the past and do not want to leave him or her, you can stay with this person for your general health care and find someone else to work with you on dealing with your fibromyalgia."

Conducting the Search

People in online fibromyalgia chat rooms cry out the same question day after day: "How do you find a doctor who can diagnose and treat fibromyalgia?" Sympathetic chatters often suggest interviewing all prospective doctors before choosing one to actually visit. But Dr.

Scherger feels that, in reality, it is rare to have the luxury of doing an extended phone interview with a doctor before you make an appointment. He believes that the best way to find a good doctor is by testimonial reputation.

"Look for people who love their doctor," he suggests. "Talk to people who have values similar to yours in what they want from a doctor. Find out who are the really good personal physicians who take a lot of time if you need it. And then find out if that doctor is willing to take on patients who might have fibromyalgia. It's not unreasonable to call a doctor's office and ask, 'Does this doctor accept patients with fibromyalgia?'" Dr. Yunus adds, "If the answer is yes, ask this second question: Can he or she do a tender point evaluation to diagnoses fibromyalgia?"

> *You may not find the right doctor right away, but the search effort is definitely worth it in the end.*

Dr. Scherger also suggests the possibility of finding a good doctor by reading the medical literature. "Keep track of who is writing the medical articles on fibromyalgia," he says. "Obviously if someone has enough interest in this topic to write about it, he or she would be a good person to go to. And this way you may find a physician right in your geographical area who is very interested in fibromyalgia who may take you on as a patient or refer you to someone known to treat and understand FMS patients."

You may not find the right doctor right away, but the search effort is definitely worth it in the end. People with fibromyalgia who have found these holistic, caring, and knowledgeable people say they feel the doctors respect them and treat them with dignity rather than with annoyance or even ridicule. Keep looking—many physicians today are not only good at diagnosing and treating fibromyalgia but do it with enthusiasm. Dr. Scherger believes, "There are a lot of doctors who find patients with this challenging problem to be very rewarding. If a doctor takes the extra time, he can turn someone's life around. As a doctor, I feel I've really done something important if I can take a patient and bring him or her from chronic illness behavior back into a productive life."

DIAGNOSING FIBROMYALGIA

So many people with fibromyalgia tell the same story of a long, drawn-out process of diagnosis that you may begin to believe this time-consuming routine of testing, testing, and more testing is to be expected. Don't believe it for a minute. Diagnosis of this illness can be swift and sure in the hands of an experienced practitioner.

FMS Is *Not* a Wastebasket Disease

Before arriving at a diagnosis of fibromyalgia, many physicians first attempt to exclude other potential diagnoses such as autoimmune disorders, digestive disorders, and musculoskeletal problems. Many diagnostic tests, including blood and urine tests, x rays, magnetic resonance imaging (MRI), and more may be performed to identify or rule out other possible diseases, ailments, disorders, and conditions with symptoms of pain and fatigue that mimic some FMS symptoms. Common suspects are lupus, Lyme disease, rheumatoid arthritis, hypothyroidism, cervical and low-back degenerative disease, sleep disorders, HIV infections, and polymyalgia rheumatica. But those who are very knowledgeable about the clinical features of fibromyalgia say this "ruling out" routine is old-fashioned and unscientific. If, after all, you test positive for one of these conditions, that doesn't mean you don't also have fibromyalgia. And if you test negative for all these conditions, that does not necessarily mean you do have fibromyalgia.

> *Those who are very knowledgeable about the clinical features of fibromyalgia say this "ruling out" routine is old-fashioned and unscientific.*

So what exactly is the point of spending all this time and money looking for what FMS is not? Dr. Yunus feels strongly that extensive testing for fibromyalgia is totally unnecessary. "Excessive testing adds to the burden of cost of medical care and contributes to the detriment of patient trust and moral, and [it] causes much inconvenience and discomfort. It's totally ridiculous to ask a patient with suspected fibromyalgia to put up with 500 pin pricks for testing and spend their time getting x rays and sitting in the waiting rooms. If a physician says the fibromyalgia can be diagnosed only by eliminating all other possible reasons for your pain and fatigue, then he or she is essentially saying that if it's nothing else—then we'll put this label on it. That makes fibromyalgia a wastebasket disease—which it is not, as clearly shown by data in the American College of Rheumatology criteria study. It is a disservice to patients to imply this."

Fibromyalgia should never be considered a disease of exclusion. Dr. Yunus emphatically states, "You will never hear this being said by the mainstream fibromyalgia researchers. You may have other concomitant ailments as well (after all, by the time you are middle aged, you are entitled to have other conditions like arthritis or such), but just as you wouldn't tell a person with osteoarthritis, 'We have to rule out 10 other causes of joint pain before we can treat you for this arthritis,' you don't need to do anything different to a person with fibromyalgia. Fibromyalgia should be diagnosed only by its own characteristic findings.

"When I give lectures on fibromyalgia, I sometimes say, 'If it walks like a duck and quacks like a duck, it is a duck.' Fibromyalgia features are so characteristic of this one condition that, just like the duck, if the symptoms of widespread pain point to fibromyalgia and it feels like fibromyalgia upon examination of tender points, it is fibromyalgia!"

If your doctor begins to order a full battery of tests for you, find out why. Fibromyalgia experts agree that tests beyond routine blood work and perhaps a test for a low thyroid hormone if a person feels excessive fatigue should be ordered only when there is evidence of a specific need—not simply to make a grand attempt to eliminate everything under the sun. "In experienced hands," says Dr. Yunus, "you do not need excessive blood or urine tests or x rays at all."

Diagnostic Procedures

When you go to a physician with symptoms of FMS, you present a perplexing problem. You look healthy. Your joints appear normal, and musculoskeletal examination indicates no objective joint swelling (even though you may feel like your joints are swollen). In addition, muscle strength, sensory functions, and reflexes are normal. If blood, urine, and x rays are unnecessary and a waste of time, how can a physician diagnose fibromyalgia? As Dr. Yunus says, "The American College of Rheumatology [ACR] criteria for fibromyalgia are disarmingly simple." Trained and experienced physicians know that fibromyalgia has distinct characteristics, as clearly identified by these criteria.

Fibromyalgia experts agree that tests beyond routine blood work and perhaps a test for a low thyroid hormone if a person feels excessive fatigue should be ordered only when there is evidence of a specific need.

In 1990, the ACR determined that fibromyalgia can be diagnosed clinically in people who have the following symptoms:

1. A history of widespread pain. The person must be experiencing pain or achiness, steady or intermittent, for at least three months. At times, the pain must have been present:

- On both the right and left sides of the body
- Both above and below the waist
- Midbody

2. Pain in at least 11 of the 18 indicated tender spots (see figure 2.1)

These 18 tender point sites used for diagnosis are symmetrically paired on each side of the body and cluster around the neck, shoulder, chest, hip, knee, and elbow regions. Many people don't know that

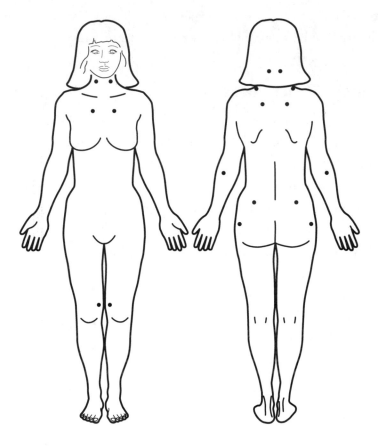

Figure 2.1—*Fibromyalgia Tender Points*

they have tender points until a doctor actually pushes on those points. Then they literally jump off the table because these areas are so tender.

Successful examination of tender points depends on knowing where to palpate and how much pressure to apply. To test the tender points, some physicians use a medical device called a *dolorimeter*. This hand held instrument measures pressure over a particular area and is used to gain data on pain. Dr. Yunus prefers to use his fingers in clinical practice to apply pressure using the tip of the thumb or index or middle finger with gradually increasing pressure until the patient re-

Speaking Out

The following quotes come from online fibromyalgia message boards:

- "Reactions to diagnosis vary. I was thrilled to finally have a name for what I knew was wrong. Others who get an immediate diagnosis may go into denial, or get very depressed, as there is so little hope of getting better."

- "When I was diagnosed with FMS, I must say I was so relieved just to put a name on this pain, fatigue, and headaches. I was relieved to know that I wasn't going to die."

- "At first I was totally elated because I knew what it was that I was dealing with, or at least the name of it. At the time I had never heard of FMS."

- "Over the past 10 years, I believe doctors have become aware of how to diagnose the illness. Some keep on top of latest developments and some do not. My doctor is quite educated on the various trials and tests."

ports that the feeling of pressure has changed to pain. He believes that the ability to find the tender points is a skill no less than the skill needed to examine the heart, the abdomen, or the lungs.

"Physicians who don't know how to do a proper physical examination to locate the tender points of fibromyalgia may feel insecure about diagnosing this problem," he says. "It has been very common for referring physicians to tell me that they find only 5 or 7 tender points, but then when I examine the patient I find all 18. When the examiner is knowledgeable and has had adequate training, there should be no problem making the diagnosis based on the presence of widespread pain and tender points."

Incomplete Fibromyalgia

Because the tender point evaluation is so critical to the diagnosis of fibromyalgia, many wonder, "What if a person has 10 but not 11 of the identified tender points? Does that mean she doesn't have fibromyalgia?" To answer this question, remember that the ACR criteria, while clinically useful, were developed primarily for uniform case classification for researchers.

The 2 percent figure given by the ACR for the percentage of the population with fibromyalgia is based only on those meeting the strict ACR criteria. The actual number of people being treated for "incomplete fibromyalgia" is much higher.

Speaking to a journalist from *Psychology Today* magazine, rheumatologist David S. Caldwell, M.D., of Duke Medical Center in Durham, North Carolina, said, "Many of us feel that if you've excluded any other disease or explanation for the symptoms, and the patient describes pain and has the other frequently associated problems, like sleep disorder, migraine headaches and so on, then regardless of whether they have the prescribed number of tender points, the diagnosis is likely to be FM."[9]

Dr. Yunus supports this view of diagnosis and presented a paper at a recent meeting of the American College of Rheumatology on patients who have what he calls "incomplete fibromyalgia." These are people who have some of the criteria necessary for a clinical diagnosis of fibromyalgia, but not all. They may have widespread pain, but not tender points; or they may have adequate tender points, but their pain may be limited to a region, such as the neck, arms, or upper back, and not exactly "widespread" as described in the criteria; or they may have both widespread pain and tender points, but fewer than the "required" 11 tender points. "These people," says Dr. Yunus, "should be treated for fibromyalgia." (It's interesting to note that the 2 percent figure given by the ACR for the percentage of the population with fibromyalgia is based only on those meeting the strict ACR criteria. The actual number of people being treated for "incomplete fibromyalgia" is much higher.)

OVERLAPPING CONDITIONS

The symptoms of fibromyalgia are similar and often confused with those of chronic fatigue syndrome (CFS) and myofascial pain syndrome (MPS). As you search through the medical literature looking for information that will help you understand why you are so tired and hurt all over, you may stop short at an article about chronic fatigue syndrome and decide, "That's exactly what I have!" But then you'll read about myofascial pain syndrome and know without a doubt, "That's what I have!" Then a book on fibromyalgia comes your way and as you read through the signs and symptoms, you're convinced that you have found the answer—or maybe not.

Fibromyalgia, CFS, and MPS are all chronic pain conditions that have overlapping symptoms. These symptoms are so much alike that some physicians and researchers believe these conditions are all varying degrees of the same problem; others believe they are three distinct conditions with overlapping symptoms. Others make no distinction between the three at all. This confusion can affect your diagnosis, so it's a good idea to know the features of each and how a doctor can try to distinguish between them.

Chronic Fatigue Syndrome

In his book *From Fatigued to Fantastic!* Dr. Jacob Teitelbaum tells us, "Chronic fatigue syndrome is a group of symptoms associated with severe, almost unrelenting fatigue. The predominant symptom is fatigue that causes a persistent and substantial reduction in activity level. Poor sleep, achiness, brain fog, increased thirst, bowel disorders, recurrent infections, and exhaustion after minimal exertion are some of the more common associated symptoms."[10]

From this typical description, you can see that the emphasis in describing CFS is on fatigue more than pain; in some cases, this distinction is all that separates CFS from FMS. A general discussion of the other symptoms of chronic fatigue syndrome sounds so similar to fibromyalgia you might swear the two were the same. As you read the following information taken from a fact sheet on the Web site of the Chronic Fatigue and Immune Dysfunction Syndrome (CFIDS) Association of America, you'll see why separating CFS from FMS is not an easy thing to do:

> Its onset is sudden but not alarming because many of the syndrome's symptoms—headache, tender lymph nodes, fatigue and weakness, muscle and joint aches, inability to concentrate—mimic those of the flu. But whereas flu symptoms usually go away in a few weeks, the symptoms of CFS do not. The onset is often hard to pinpoint. Sometimes it seems to be triggered by an acute infection such as a cold, bronchitis, hepatitis, mononucleosis, or an intestinal bug. In others, the syndrome develops more gradually, with no clear triggering event. Often a patient reports that the illness emerged during a period of high stress. No specific treatments exist, but symptomatic treatment still can be quite helpful.[11]

Doesn't that sound like a description of fibromyalgia? However, despite this similarity, the criteria for diagnosing CFS that distinguishes it from other ailments were established in 1994 by a joint committee including members of the U.S. Centers for Disease Control and Prevention and the National Institutes of Health. This set of criteria states that the symptoms of CFS include unexplained persistent or relapsing chronic fatigue. It specifies that this fatigue is not the kind that results from ongoing exertion, is not substantially alleviated by rest, and results in substantial reduction in previous levels of occupational, educational, social, or personal activities.

The emphasis in describing CFS is on fatigue more than pain; in some cases, this distinction is all that separates CFS from FMS.

The criteria further states that, along with fatigue, a person with CFS will have four or more of the following symptoms during six or more consecutive months:

- Substantial impairment in short-term memory or concentration
- Sore throat
- Tender lymph nodes
- Muscle pain
- Multijoint pain without joint swelling or redness
- Headaches of a new type, pattern, or severity
- Nonrefreshing sleep
- Postexertional malaise lasting more than 24 hours

Using this criteria you can see that people diagnosed with FMS might certainly also have CFS, or they may indeed be one and the same thing. To add to the confusion, Leslie A. Aaron, Ph.D., MPH, from the Department of Medicine at Harborview Medical Center in Seattle, Washington, says that although there are specific, published criteria for fibromyalgia and chronic fatigue syndrome, which diagnosis you get can depend on what kind of physician you go to. "People who are knowledgeable in this field competently apply the medical criteria to their patients, but many physicians do not rely on the criteria," she says. "They have a less formal way of distinguishing between these pain syndromes depending on what they are most familiar with. If, for example, a physician has received training from someone who frequently works with fibromyalgia patients, he or she will interpret the overlapping symptoms to be fibromyalgia. To make a general statement, it seems that a rheumatologist is more likely to diagnose fibromyalgia and a general internist looking at the same symptoms may diagnose chronic fatigue."

This concern over the lax application of published criteria for FMS and CFS is shared by Laurence Bradley, Ph.D., professor of medicine in the Division of Clinical Immunology and Rheumatology at the University of Alabama, Birmingham, who is nationally renown for his work with fibromyalgia and CFS. He feels that part of the problem with trying to separate these pain syndromes into neat and separate disease states is that some medical and lay literature don't distinguish between these syndromes at all. "While there are agreed-upon classification criteria for each one," he says, "there are variations in how investigators apply the criteria, and they don't always report in their samples how many people met the criteria for one or both."

To separate the fibromyalgia patients from the chronic fatigue syndrome patients some researchers require fibromyalgia patients to have more than seven tender points and chronic fatigue patients to have no more than seven tender points. Yet, as mentioned earlier, some physicians will diagnose fibromyalgia in patients who have widespread pain but very few (certainly fewer than seven) tender points. Again, the confusion lies in the fact that there is no agreed-on way to distinguish between fibromyalgia and chronic fatigue syndrome, so we have variations among investigators.

But Dr. Bradley admits that even when physicians and researchers carefully follow the published criteria guidelines, much confusion still persists:

> The main problem in separating these two syndromes," he says, "is that we don't know whether chronic fatigue and fibromyalgia are variations on a spectrum of pain and fatigue-type disorders, or whether they really represent distinct entities. Right now our research program is trying to determine the pathophysiological similarities and differences between people with these syndromes. We have an ongoing protocol that is looking at changes in functional brain activity in response to painful or noxious stimulation in patients who meet the criteria only for fibromyalgia versus patients who meet the criteria only for chronic fatigue syndrome. We think that by examining these two distinct groups, we can better identify the brain patterns that may differentiate between them.

Dr. Aaron states that, currently, the tender-point exam and associated criteria for FMS and CFS are the gold standards for differentiating between the disorders. She says, "If a physician says, 'You have widespread pain, fatigue, and tenderness in 11 out of 18 tender point sites, and, therefore, I am diagnosing fibromyalgia,' you can be assured that the diagnosis has been made correctly." But you may have to push to get this kind of precise information. When your doctor says that you have one of these pain syndromes, you can't be shy about asking how he or she arrived at that diagnosis. Drs. Bradley and Aaron agree that people have to ask the person who gives them a diagnosis of fibromyalgia to explain the criteria that were used to make the diagnosis and how the other pain syndromes were ruled out. Dr. Bradley says, "Your doctor should say to you something like, 'Here are the published, standard criteria, and here's where you fall within that spectrum.'"

Keep in mind that having a definitive diagnosis of fibromyalgia does not rule out the possibility that you have chronic fatigue syndrome also. Dr. Aaron and her research colleagues have identified several studies that confirm the overlapping symptoms of fibromyalgia and chronic fatigue syndrome. They report that an estimated 20 to 70 percent of people with FMS also meet criteria for CFS.[12] A study of 3,395 people in England and Canada verifies what many people and physicians have noticed about this overlap: When an individual has both FMS and CFS, the symptoms of both are more severe and disruptive of daily life.[13] So, if you have been diagnosed with fibromyalgia but feel you might also have CFS, don't be afraid to talk to your doctor about that possibility.

> *Ask the person who gives you a diagnosis of fibromyalgia to explain the criteria that were used to make the diagnosis and how the other pain syndromes were ruled out.*

Myofascial Pain Syndrome

Myofascial pain syndrome (MPS) has been defined by Dr. Yunus in his article "Fibromyalgia Syndrome and Myofascial Pain Syndrome" as a regional pain syndrome accompanied by trigger points. He notes that some people with MPS also experience symptoms of stiff joints, poor sleep, fatigue, numbness of the extremities, nausea, and constipation.[14] This description certainly sounds similar to a description of fibromyalgia, except for two points that are easily glossed over if one is not careful:

1. Myofascial pain syndrome causes *regional* pain, whereas fibromyalgia causes widespread pain. (Be careful if you come across the term *regional fibromyalgia;* it is an incorrect label for MPS.)

2. Trigger points accompany myofascial pain syndrome, whereas tender points accompany fibromyalgia.

> *Tender points hurt only when pressed and only at the tender point site. Trigger points hurt without touching them, and when they are pressed, the pain shoots to other areas in the body.*

The overwhelming characteristic of fibromyalgia is long-standing pain at defined tender points, which are not the same as the trigger points of MPS. Tender points hurt only when pressed and only at the tender point site. Trigger points hurt without touching them, and when they are pressed, the pain shoots to other areas in the body (called *referred pain*). Devin J. Starlanyl and Mary Ellen Copeland talk about these trigger points of MPS in their book *Fibromyalgia and Chronic Myofascial Pain Syndrome: A Survival Manual:*

Trigger points seem to form throughout life as a response to many things that happen to our bodies. Overuse, repetitive motion trauma, bruises, strains, joint problems, etc. Pain creates a neuromuscular response, and the muscle around the pain site tightens, "guarding" the hurt area. When muscles are in a state of sustained tension, they are working, even if you're not. A working muscle needs more nutrition and oxygen, and produces more waste, than a muscle at rest. This creates an area starved for food and oxygen, and loaded with toxic waste—a trigger point.[15]

This is quite different from tender points that many people with fibromyalgia do not even know they have.

Despite these differences, Dr. Bradley believes that separating fibromyalgia from myofascial pain syndrome is a very difficult task.

FMS or MPS?

The conditions of FMS and MPS definitely overlap, but there are some primary differences that may help you distinguish one from the other:

- The musculoskeletal pain of FMS is widespread.
- The musculoskeletal pain of MPS is regional.
- The tender points of FMS are widespread and multiple.
- The trigger points of MPS are regional and few.

"The pain of myofascial pain syndrome is typically more localized than the widespread pain of fibromyalgia, but it's a very fine line that differentiates the tender points of fibromyalgia from the trigger points of myofascial pain syndrome. Although it's not impossible to separate one from the other, it's very hard to do."

Adding to the difficulty of separating these two syndromes is the fact that many physicians and researchers now recognize that some people have both the tender points of FMS and the trigger points of MPS, leading to what Dr. Starlanyl calls FMS/MPS complex. If, in addition to the fibromyalgic tender points that your doctor finds, you also have what may be knotty, trigger points in one localized area, ask your doctor to examine you for myofascial pain syndrome as well. Untreated MPS can become a chronic pain condition.

Leslie A. Aaron, Ph.D., MPH, of the Department of Medicine at Harborview Medical Center in Seattle, Washington, adds:

There are a lot of researchers and physicians who lump FMS, CFS, and MPS together as the same thing. They don't feel separating one from the other makes any difference to the method of treatment, so they don't distinguish between them in diagnosis. It remains to be seen whether the research will reveal specific effective treatments for individual disorders. But I think it's important to get to the bottom of exactly what is happening to you. Getting a correct label for what you have and a basis for understanding it is important to the recovery and management process of any chronic condition.

A Possible Connection

Dr. Yunus believes that fibromyalgia, chronic fatigue syndrome, and myofascial pain syndrome are overlapping conditions but also that they are all part of a spectrum of conditions he calls *central sensitivity syndromes* (CSS). (He also includes irritable bowel syndrome, headaches, and restless legs syndrome in this spectrum.) The basis of this collection is the fact that these disorders all share several features, including:

- Pain
- Fatigue
- Poor sleep patterns
- Hyperalgesic state (exaggerated response to normally painful stimulus)
- Irritable bowel
- Headaches
- Absence of "hard" physical signs and pathological changes in the peripheral tissues
- Lack of a specific laboratory test for diagnosis
- Presence of a neuroendocrine dysfunction, which is different from those seen in psychiatric diseases

In addition, all three conditions are found predominantly in females between the ages of 30 and 60 and can be triggered by trauma, infection, or mechanical stresses.

Dr. Yunus feels that central sensitivity syndromes such as FMS, CFS, and MPS present physicians with a paradigm for diagnosis that separates them from (1) those illnesses and conditions that have been

Fibromyalgia Survey

The following list shows the percentage of people in the Ferguson survey who reported having these coexisting or preexisting diagnoses:

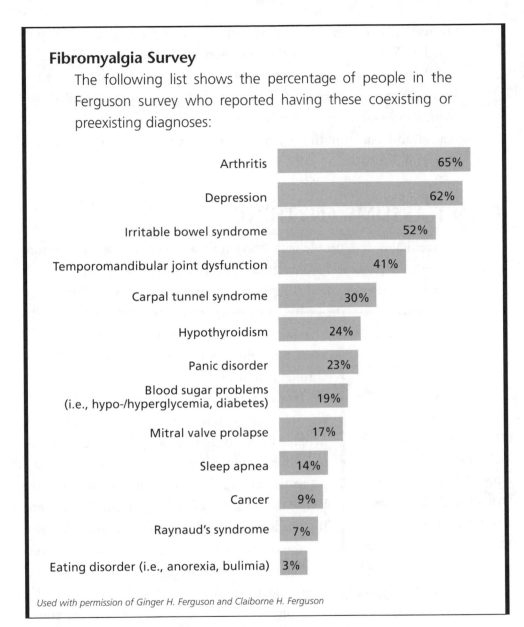

Arthritis	65%
Depression	62%
Irritable bowel syndrome	52%
Temporomandibular joint dysfunction	41%
Carpal tunnel syndrome	30%
Hypothyroidism	24%
Panic disorder	23%
Blood sugar problems (i.e., hypo-/hyperglycemia, diabetes)	19%
Mitral valve prolapse	17%
Sleep apnea	14%
Cancer	9%
Raynaud's syndrome	7%
Eating disorder (i.e., anorexia, bulimia)	3%

Used with permission of Ginger H. Ferguson and Claiborne H. Ferguson

called "organic" and are identified by physical abnormalities such as degenerative joint disease, inflammatory bowel diseases, or cancer and (2) psychiatric diseases such as depression or anxiety disorders. This "third paradigm" proposed by Dr. Yunus is based instead on a dysfunction of the central nervous system and the interacting endocrine system that regulates pain, sleep, and fatigue (as explained in chapter 1). Dr. Yunus states that the common glue that binds FMS, CFS, MPS, and other similar syndromes is a dysfunction of the central nervous system characterized by neuron hypersensitivity (called *central sensitivity*). If this premise proves to be true, research into the cause and cure for these syndromes can proceed in a unified and hopeful direction.

DON'T ASSUME ANYTHING

Once diagnosed, people with fibromyalgia tend to chalk off all future aches and pains as FMS related. This is a dangerous assumption. If you have other conditions commonly found in people with FMS, such as osteoarthritis, rheumatoid arthritis, or disc herniation, these problems must be treated separately. They cannot be lumped into the FMS pile and ignored, just because you have a chronic pain disorder.

> *If you have other conditions commonly found in people with FMS, such as osteoarthritis, rheumatoid arthritis, or disc herniation, these problems must be treated separately.*

If you feel new pain that is chronic but "different," don't assume it isn't anything new. Even people with fibromyalgia get kidney stones, pneumonia, and cancer. Ask yourself, "Would I go to the doctor for this pain if I did not have FMS?" If the answer is yes, then call your doctor. If your doctor should imply or insinuate that you call too often, then it's time to find a new doctor.

When all is said and done about the difficulties of diagnosing fibromyalgia, the fact remains that if you find a trained and experienced physician, the telltale symptoms of fibromyalgia can be easily detected. Before you begin a treatment regime as described in the following chapters, make sure you feel confident that you have received the correct diagnosis.

CHAPTER 3

Medical Treatments

SADLY, THERE IS no guaranteed cure for fibromyalgia. No treatment, drug, or therapy is certain to make it go away. Some patients do recover with treatment, lifestyle changes, or the body's ability to heal itself. We can hope that one of the many research projects being conducted today to find this cure will soon make the outlook more hopeful. In the meantime, the following information will help you better understand the medical treatments your doctor may prescribe to give you relief from your chronic symptoms and to help you improve or recover.

If you join a fibromyalgia support group, or go to online chats, or talk to a friend or relative who also has fibromyalgia, you'll quickly find that your treatment program may be quite different from everybody else's. That's because the treatment for fibromyalgia must be tailored specifically to each person's needs. Since fibromyalgia is a syndrome, by its very definition it is a collection of symptoms that vary from one person to another. In this case, the treatment for these different symptoms is complicated by the fact that even the severity and frequency of symptoms vary from one person to another. Some people with fibromyalgia have mild symptoms and need very little treatment. Others suffer flare-ups that require immediate and intensive treatment, but then subside,

No Simple Bug

People want fibromyalgia to be like pneumonia. They want there to be a bug that causes it, and they want to think that if they can kill that bug, the illness and its resultant features will no longer be there. But fibromyalgia is not like pneumonia, and it's unlikely that any one clear-cut cause will be found.

—DON GOLDENBERG, M.D.

and treatment must be adjusted again. Still others suffer persistent, unrelenting, and often debilitating symptoms that need constant medical supervision.

Muhammad B. Yunus, M.D., acknowledges this complex state in his article "Fibromyalgia Syndrome: Is There Any Effective Therapy?" He says, "Many different factors interact to cause symptoms, and their relative importance varies from patient to patient. Consequently, 'one-size treatment' does not fit all patients."[1]

Fortunately, all medical researchers and physicians agree on one fact: Although most people with fibromyalgia continue to have chronic pain, appropriate management with a *multifaceted* and *individualized* treatment approach can improve function and quality of life. Without exception, successful treatment programs include a mix of physician-directed medical approaches, as well as individualized and self-directed programs that combine therapies such as exercise, relaxation strategies, help with sleep, diet changes, psychotherapy, and a wide range of complementary and alternative treatments.

This book explores the treatment therapies most commonly recommended by the nation's top fibromyalgia experts. Your doctor may have suggestions not found here that may work for you, but in addition, he or she will surely agree with a multifaceted approach that includes parts and pieces of these four therapies explained in the following chapters:

1. Medical treatments

2. Exercise and stress reduction strategies

3. Mind-body healing techniques, including cognitive and behavioral therapies

4. Complementary and alternative treatments, such as massage and acupuncture

THE ROOT OF FMS DISCOMFORT

Education is the first line of treatment for anyone with fibromyalgia. Because this is a complex syndrome that has no single protocol of treatment, your doctor may try a little of this and a little of that, hoping to find something that works for you. In this kind of trial-and-error approach, you can easily lose track of why you are doing what

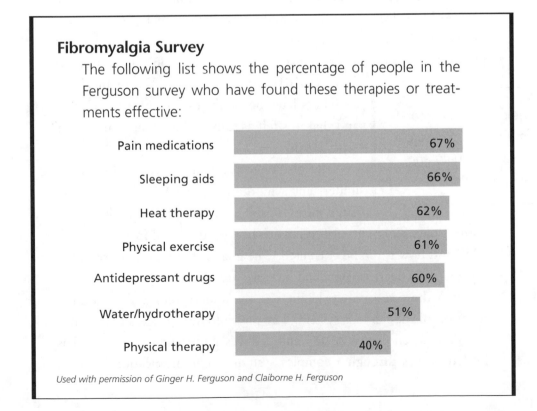

Fibromyalgia Survey

The following list shows the percentage of people in the Ferguson survey who have found these therapies or treatments effective:

Therapy	Percentage
Pain medications	67%
Sleeping aids	66%
Heat therapy	62%
Physical exercise	61%
Antidepressant drugs	60%
Water/hydrotherapy	51%
Physical therapy	40%

Used with permission of Ginger H. Ferguson and Claiborne H. Ferguson

you're doing if you don't understand the reasons for the strategies you will try. This section will give you a brief primer on how the body regulates pain and sleep and how treatment therapies attempt to affect these natural processes. This information will help you have more control over your health.

Is Chronic Pain *Real* Pain?

The sensation of pain has an important function: It lets us know when something is wrong, and it insists that the problem be rectified immediately. In fact, pain itself is not a problem at all but merely the identifier of one. Without pain signals, we would not quickly remove our hand from a burning flame and would suffer severe, perhaps irreparable, damage. We need the sensation of pain to keep us alert to physical and medical problems. As smoke detectors sense the fire, so, too, is acute pain only the detector, not the fire.

But chronic pain like the pain of fibromyalgia is different. It is a wayward fire siren—a relentless and unforgiving signal of distress, refusing to silence even when the fire is out. Often, it is pain without physical signs of injury or damage. It is pain that won't show itself on x rays, MRIs, or blood tests. Yet medical researchers have no doubt that it is very real pain and that it is felt as fully and acutely as any other type of pain.

> *The goal in the treatment of fibromyalgia is to decrease pain and increase function.*

The challenge for medical researchers is to understand why the pain of FMS is chronic and often unresponsive to treatment—why the body's natural pain signal process seems to be dysfunctional in people with FMS and how it can be corrected. The goal in the treatment of fibromyalgia is to decrease pain and increase function.

First these researchers begin with the understanding that pain is a function of the nervous system. The physiological process that amplifies pain when injury occurs and reduces pain when the injury has healed occurs through a complex system of communication between the brain and the spinal cord. The messenger units that carry the body's internal communications are biochemical substances called *neurotransmitters*.

Ken Giuffre, M.D., president of Trilobot Institute for Applied Cognitive Research in New Jersey and author of the book *The Care and Feeding of the Brain*, explains that the migration of the neurotransmitters to the brain is initiated by small nerve cells, called *nocioceptors*, that are located all over the body:

> When the nocioceptors sense physical danger, they send two signals to the brain," he says. "One piece of information is sent directly and quickly to the brain to identify the location of the danger and determine what action is needed to rectify the situation. The second message transmits a neurotransmitter, known as substance P, on a longer and less direct path up the spine to the brain cell neurons. The neurons identify substance P with their antenna-like structures and connect with the neurotransmitter in a lock-and-key fashion. The neuron then fires a biochemical mixture that contains more substance P, which proceeds to find more receptive neurons; the result is a chain reaction that causes the sensation of pain.

You may have witnessed these two pain signals at work in your own body. Have you ever cut yourself badly with a knife, quickly dropped the knife in horror, and then looked at a gaping wound in your hand, realizing that you haven't yet felt pain? This happens because the nocioceptor shot the danger message to the brain to drop the knife and stop the damage to the hand—this was the more urgent message. The body's first priority is self-preservation; in a case like this, your body first uses its energy to remove the danger. Then substance P arrives a few seconds later and the sensation of pain soon follows.

The arrival of substance P is slightly delayed because it must first pass through a "gate" at the bottom of the spinal cord. This gate must open to allow substance P access to the brain. As the brain is flooded with the pain signal, it releases other neurotransmitters to help reduce the pain sensation. In a healthy person, these chemicals (such as serotonin, norepinephrine, and dopamine) regulate substance P; as the injury heals, they reduce the levels of substance P and thus the perception of pain.

In chronic pain states, the process works the same with one exception. For unknown reasons, substance P is allowed to bring pain messages continually to the brain, and the pain inhibitory mechanisms do not work as they should. This unbalanced state of neurotransmitters has been the focus of much FMS research. I. Jon Russell, M.D., Ph.D., of the University of Texas at San Antonio, has found that the levels of substance P in the spinal fluid of people with FMS is three times greater than the levels found in healthy people.[2] And other research has found that the concentrations of three brain chemicals that regulate levels of substance P—dopamine, norepinephrine, and serotonin—are abnormally low in people with FMS.[3]

For all these reasons, many of the medications used to treat FMS work to regulate the levels of these pain system regulators.

Why Deep Sleep Won't Come

As mentioned in chapter 1, approximately 75 percent of people with FMS have sleep disorders.[4] If, regardless of the number of hours you sleep, you wake in the morning feeling tired and unrefreshed and

---

A Classic Study

A classic study by Harvey Moldofsky, M.D., from the University of Ontario, Canada, created the symptoms of FMS by depriving healthy student volunteers of their sleep. Within 4 days, almost all of them had symptoms indistinguishable from FMS. The only ones who did not were the well-conditioned, high-performance athletes who took a few days longer before they showed these symptoms.[5]

then drag yourself through the day, you probably have a sleep disorder that needs to be treated as part of your fibromyalgia management program.

Some experts in this field of medicine are convinced that fibromyalgia is in fact caused by a sleep dysfunction. In his book *From Fatigued to Fantastic!* Dr. Jacob Teitelbaum says, "Fibromyalgia is basically a sleep disorder characterized by many tender knots in the muscles." Dr. Joseph E. Scherger, too, believes sleep dysfunction is at least partly to blame for the symptoms of FMS. "In my more than 10 years of working with FMS," says Dr. Scherger, "I have not yet found one patient who can tell me he wakes up in the morning rested after a good night's sleep. People with fibromyalgia tend to be people who are carrying around so much tension in their body that is not getting released by restful sleep. The tension builds up, and soon they find themselves dealing with the symptoms of fibromyalgia."

Not everyone agrees with this view of the syndrome, but whether sleep dysfunction is the cause of FMS or not, there is no question among leading medical authorities that lack of deep sleep is a major contributing factor to the symptoms of fibromyalgia and therefore sleep therapy needs to be a part of the treatment program.

> *There is no question among leading medical authorities that lack of deep sleep is a major contributing factor to the symptoms of fibromyalgia and therefore sleep therapy needs to be a part of the treatment program.*

Understanding Sleep Stages

We can thank the invention of the electroencephalogram (EEG) in 1935 for this insight into the sleep problems of people with FMS. Before this invention, it was believed that sleep was largely static and filled with inactivity. But the EEG allowed scientists to record the electrical activity of the brain and determine that discrete brain wave patterns occur in regular cycles. An irregularity in these cycles can cause many of the physical problems associated with FMS. To understand those problems, let's take a quick look at how sleep is structured throughout the night.

Humans experience two types of sleep: non-REM (usually pronounced "non-rem" and written *NREM*) and REM sleep. NREM sleep is divided into four stages. During NREM sleep, you lie quietly as your brain emits slow, regular waves. Depending on the amount of sleep you get every night, you can experience anywhere from four to six sleep cycles. Each cycle lasts about 90 minutes and contains up to four sleep stages and a REM period.

Falling asleep is like descending a staircase, with each stage of sleep becoming deeper than the previous one. At the onset of sleep you enter the first stage. This is a transitional period between wakefulness and sleep lasting only about 3 to 5 minutes. Alpha waves, emitted by the brain and associated with relaxed wakefulness, disappear and are replaced by slower, more regular theta waves. In addition, body temperature begins to drop and muscles begin to relax. Because some sections of the brain have fallen asleep and others are still awake during stage 1, information from the environment is still being processed. Therefore, you are still easily aroused. It is not unusual for you to be awakened by a *myoclonic jerk*—a muscle contraction of the arm, leg, or entire body.

> *F*alling asleep is like descending a staircase, with each stage of sleep becoming deeper than the previous one.

After the rather brief stage 1 transition period between wakefulness and sleep, you enter into the slightly deeper sleep of stage 2. This sleep lasts about 30 to 40 minutes. More time is spent in stage 2 sleep than in any other stage—about 50 percent of the night's total sleep time.

Stages 3 and 4, the last two stages of NREM sleep, are usually grouped together. During these two stages, brain wave activity slows down. Sleep becomes very deep as your brain emits high, wide delta waves. Because of the type of brain waves emitted, stage 3 and stage 4 sleep are often referred to as "deep delta sleep." Only 20 to 25 percent of the night's sleep is spent in these stages. During stages 3 and 4, heart rate and breathing become very regular. In addition, you become less sensitive to light and sound and are therefore difficult to awaken. This delta sleep is valuable in restoring and revitalizing the body.

After stage 4 sleep is complete, you ascend through stages 3 and 2. Rather than going back into stage 1 and waking, however, you experience the night's first period of REM sleep. REM sleep is the period during which dreams occur. During REM (an acronym of *rapid eye movement*), your eyes move back and forth quickly beneath your eyelids as your mind dreams. Your heart rate becomes slightly irregular, and your breathing becomes very irregular, as you experience bursts of eye movement activity and muscle twitches. About one-quarter of the night is spent in REM sleep; each REM period becomes increasingly longer until toward the end of the night, when they can last as long as an hour.

At the conclusion of the first REM period, the night's first sleep cycle comes to an end and you begin the second cycle of sleep. This cycle begins with stage 2 sleep and follows the same pattern as the first cycle. Once again you descend into the deepest stages of sleep and finish the cycle with a REM period. In adults, the later sleep cycles lack delta sleep. Stage 4 sleep disappears by the third cycle, and stage 3 sleep disappears by the fourth cycle. The last part of the night you alternate between stage 2 sleep and REM sleep. Because of the lack of delta sleep in the later cycles, the most restorative effects of a night's sleep are accomplished during the first 3 to 5 hours of sleep.[6] If you are easily awakened by the slightest noise in the middle of the night (when you should be in deep stage 4 sleep), you may not be getting enough of this restorative sleep, and this fact can be contributing to, aggravating, or even causing your fibromyalgia.

> *Because of the type of brain waves emitted, stage 3 and stage 4 sleep are often referred to as "deep delta sleep." This delta sleep is valuable in restoring and revitalizing the body.*

Sleeping (or Not) with FMS

It is during stage 4 sleep that the sleep disorder closely associated with fibromyalgia occurs. Researcher Dr. Harvey Moldofsky found that FMS patients can often fall asleep without much trouble, but their deep level (stage 4) sleep was constantly interrupted by bursts of awake-like brain activity. They can't stay in this stage of sleep for the amount of time necessary to gain its restorative benefits.

*M*any of the medications frequently prescribed to treat the chronic fatigue and pain of FMS work to increase serotonin and norepinephrine.

This sleep disorder is called the *alpha-EEG anomaly*. Because many people with fibromyalgia have this sleep problem, many believe that lack of deep delta sleep may cause, or at the very least aggravate, the pain of FMS. It is during this stage that the brain releases the growth hormone somatotropin. This hormone stimulates growth in children and adolescents, but it has an important function in adults as well. It repairs the microtraumas that occur to our muscles each day as we walk, bend, lift, and stretch. It also helps remove the lactic acid and other substances that build up in muscles during exertion. Without an adequate supply of somatotropin, we feel increased muscle pain and a decrease in repair to damaged tissues—both contributing to the daily pain of FMS.

One possible reason for this disruption of normal sleep is a low supply of two brain chemicals (neurotransmitters) that regulate deep-level sleep: serotonin and norepinephrine. Concentrations of these brain chemicals are abnormally low in people who have FMS. (It's interesting to note that these two chemicals are also needed to reduce pain!) This sleep problem is another reason why many of the medications frequently prescribed to treat the chronic fatigue and pain of FMS work to increase serotonin and norepinephrine.

TREATING FMS WITH MEDICATION

Your doctor has many medications to choose from when treating the pain, fatigue, and sleep problems associated with fibromyalgia. But prescribing for fibromyalgia is a complex ordeal because no medication has been approved by the Food and Drug Administration (FDA) for treatment of this illness. Your doctor has to borrow drugs approved for the treatment of other diseases in a mix-and-match regimen. She'll take a little of this for the pain, a little of that for the fatigue, and throw in a little of something else to improve sleep problems. The medications that are most commonly used for their track record of effectiveness are ones that raise levels of serotonin and norepinephrine to ease pain and promote sleep, ones that stimulate the central nervous system to reduce fatigue, ones that relax muscles to smooth tight knotted musculature, and ones that block pain messages traveling through the central nervous system. The specific ones discussed in this chapter include nonsteroidal anti-inflammatory drugs, antidepressants, muscle relaxants, sleeping pills, narcotic analgesics, and trigger point injections. Because treatment options for FMS are as varied as the many people who have it, you should have a clear understanding of these options to find the one that is best for you.

> *No* medication has been approved by the FDA for treatment of this illness. Your doctor has to borrow drugs approved for the treatment of other diseases in a mix-and-match regimen.

Note: The general descriptions of the various drugs used to treat fibromyalgia offered in this chapter are adapted from the online U.S. National Library of Medicine. Your doctor may have additional information regarding the specific drug he or she prescribes.

Nonsteroidal Anti-Inflammatory Drugs

Nonsteroidal anti-inflammatory drugs (NSAIDs) are used to relieve symptoms such as swelling, stiffness, and joint pain that are caused by inflammation. They are commonly prescribed for the chronic pain of arthritis (rheumatism), but some physicians recommend them also for the pain of fibromyalgia.

NSAIDs include common brand names such as Advil, Aleve, Anaprox, Bayer Select Ibuprofen Pain Relief Formula Caplets,

Daypro, Excedrin IB, Motrin, Nuprin, Pamprin, Relafen, Lodine, and Voltaren. These medications commonly contain aspirin, ibuprofen, or naproxen.

Aspirin, the 200-milligram strength of ibuprofen, and the 220-milligram strength of naproxen are available without a prescription. But the other NSAIDs and other strengths of ibuprofen and naproxen are available only with a medical doctor's prescription.

Although NSAIDs are frequently suggested as the first line of attack on the pain of FMS, unfortunately they have not been found to be very effective. Muhammad B. Yunus, M.D., professor of medicine at the University of Illinois College of Medicine, conducted a study that found no clear benefits of using ibuprofen in the treatment of fibromyalgia.[7] Similarly, Robert Godfrey, M.D., has stated in his article in the *Archives of Internal Medicine*, "Most patients with FMS are referred to a rheumatologist because treatment with nonsteroidal anti-inflammatory drugs has been ineffective. The consensus of most rheumatologists and authors is that, when used alone, nonsteroidal anti-inflammatory drugs are of little if any benefit in treating FMS."[8] So if your doctor says, "Take some Advil and see if that helps," be sure to ask why. It is very clear that the pain of FMS is not caused by inflammation and will not respond to NSAID treatment.

> *It is very clear that the pain of FMS is not caused by inflammation and will not respond to NSAID treatment.*

However, sometimes NSAIDs can work in combination with other medications to reduce the pain of FMS. So if your doctor says, "Take an Advil along with this prescription for an antidepressant," he may be on to something that will work. It seems that NSAIDs can boost the power of tricyclic antidepressants. (See the section later in this chapter called "Combination Therapy" for more information.)

Your doctor may also prescribe a NSAID to treat other conditions you may have along with FMS. If you also have rheumatoid arthritis, osteoarthritis, bursitis, tendonitis, costochondritis, endometriosis, or another condition that causes pain from inflammation, NSAIDs may be part of your medical regimen.

Precautions While Using NSAIDs

If you do find pain relief from NSAIDs, talk to your doctor about how to take them safely over time. These medications are known to cause damage to your stomach and digestive tract that can lead to ulcers when used for a long time or in large doses. If you take this medicine for more than 1 or 2 months or in large amounts, ask about other forms of treatment that might help reduce the amount of this medicine that you take or the length of treatment. Or ask your doctor about the latest types of NSAIDs that are COX-2 inhibitors (such as Celebrex and Vioxx)—they do not cause gastric upset.[9]

Switching to Celebrex has made a world of difference for Cheryl. Cheryl is a science writer in the media relations department of a major university who was diagnosed with fibromyalgia 5 years ago. Because Cheryl also has osteoarthritis, her doctor put her on a regimen of 12 ibuprofen tablets a day. But after a year had passed with only intermittent pain relief, she began to experience major stomach problems and was ready to quit using NSAIDs completely. Then her doctor gave her the COX-2 inhibitor called Celebrex. "I think these COX-2 inhibitors are just great," she says. "I've been on them only a few months, and already I'm now able to run around after my grandchildren, and I feel better than I have in years."

Ultram: A Commonly Used Analgesic

The prescription analgesic Ultram (tramadol) is often prescribed to treat the pain of FMS. This drug is a weak opioid that acts like an antidepressant to increase levels of both serotonin and norepinephrine. The effects of tramadol are similar to those of narcotic analgesics, but it is not a controlled substance and can be prescribed without the paperwork involved with true narcotics.

A study of 100 patients revealed that only 27 percent of the patients who took tramadol withdrew from the study because of inadequate pain relief.[10] Robert Bennett, M.D., of Oregon Health Sciences University in Portland, Oregon, who has approximately 6,000 patients, has reported in *Fibromyalgia Network Newsletter*, "In my practice, I have found that Ultram is particularly effective in 60 to 70 percent of my fibromyalgic patients."[11] Dr. Charles Lapp, M.D., agrees. In this same article he states: "After addressing sleep, the next most important symptom to manage is pain. When conservative measures are not enough, Ultram is an excellent choice for pain control. Efficacy is good, and habituation is unusual except in those with previous addiction problems. Ultram increases serotonin, which may also help a person with FMS feel somewhat better."[12]

In his article on FMS published in *Consultant*, Dr. Yunus also agrees, saying, "My colleagues and I have used tramadol with impressive results in some patients with FMS. This unique analgesic has its effects on opioid receptors, and it inhibits the reuptake of both serotonin and noradrenaline. Because of tramadol's weak affinity for [Mu]-opioid receptors, addiction is rare."[13]

Precautions While Using Ultram

Tramadol may cause some people to become drowsy, dizzy, or lightheaded. Nausea or vomiting may also occur, especially after the first couple of doses. Lying down for a while may also help relieve some of these side effects. However, if nausea or vomiting continues, check with your doctor.[14]

Antidepressants

How insulting! You walk into you doctor's office with complaints of pain, and she sends you out with a prescription for an antidepressant. "I'm not depressed," you may complain. "I'm in pain!" Hopefully, your doctor will explain that this prescription, although certainly helpful to

Ask Your Doctor

When you receive a prescription for medication, ask your doctor the following questions:

- What category drug is this—antidepressant, muscle relaxant, sedative, analgesic?
- Can I safely take this drug along with other prescription drugs I'm taking?
- What are the possible side effects?
- What should I do if I experience these side effects?
- How long before I notice any results?
- How long can I stay on this medication?
- Are there any over-the-counter drugs I should not take (such as cold or allergy medications) while I'm on this prescription drug?

the 30 percent of people who have clinical depression along with their fibromyalgia, is often prescribed "off label" to help reduce the symptoms of FMS. In doses much smaller than those used to treat depression, the tricyclic antidepressants and trazodone improve stage 4 sleep and help people with FMS get the deep, restorative sleep they lack. Pain relief and renewed energy often soon follow. However, they may also result in such unpleasant side effects as dry mouth or drowsiness.[15]

Tricyclic Antidepressants

Tricyclic antidepressants affect the symptoms of pain, fatigue, and sleeplessness by acting on neurotransmitters such as serotonin, norepinephrine, and histamines in varying degrees. It is thought that they may also increase the level of the body's natural painkillers (endorphins) in the brain.

Some tricyclic antidepressants commonly used to treat FMS are amitriptyline (Elavil, Endep), doxepin (Adapin, Sinequan), and nortriptyline (Aventyl, Pamelor). Trazodone (Desyrel) is another drug commonly used to treat FMS that has properties similar to tricyclic antidepressants. These medicines are available only with your doctor's prescription.

> *Drugs like tricyclic antidepressants and trazodone improve stage 4 sleep and help people with FMS get the deep, restorative sleep they lack. Pain relief and renewed energy often soon follow.*

After reviewing nine studies on tricyclics, researchers led by Lesley M. Arnold, M.D., associate professor of psychiatry at the University of Cincinnati College of Medicine, report that 25 to 37 percent of people with fibromyalgia showed some improvements when treated with tricyclic antidepressants including amitriptyline (i.e., Elavil). The largest improvement was associated with measures of sleep quality; the most modest improvement was found in measures of stiffness and tenderness.[16]

It is believed that tricyclic antidepressants may achieve these results by slowing down the reabsorption of serotonin and possibly norepinephrine. The findings have been supported by other studies and through anecdotal patient reports. Dr. Yunus advises physicians, "Tricyclic antidepressants, taken in low doses (10 to 50 mg after supper or at bedtime), are generally effective. Zolpidem (10 mg at bedtime) has been reported to improve sleep as well as daytime energy in a controlled study." He adds that he calls these drugs "'serotonin builders' rather than 'antidepressants,' because most patients with FMS are not depressed and feel hesitant, even indignant, about taking an antidepressant."[17]

But tricyclic antidepressants may not work for everybody. In a study published in the *Journal of Rheumatology*, Glenn McCain, M.D., of Charlotte, North Carolina, says, "Amitriptyline doesn't seem as effective in treating patients who have had the chronic symptoms of FMS for more than five years. Also, this drug does not appear to work as well on patients who are experiencing a comparatively high level of pain."[18] And Dr. Godfrey agrees as he cautions, "It is very important to remember that, at best, only about 50 percent of patients with FMS can be expected to show a striking response to tricyclic antidepressants. More patients will get more modest and only partial relief, while a small, significant, but unfortunate group will show little or no response to any of the antidepressants."[19] Still, tricyclic antidepressants are a popular line of treatment many physicians try as they begin to explore the possibilities.

Precautions While Using Tricyclic Antidepressants

You should have frequent medical checkups while taking tricyclic antidepressants. Between visits, monitor your health by remembering that the undesirable side effects of tricyclic antidepressants can include constipation, dry mouth, drowsiness, weight gain, dizziness, blurred vision, urinary retention, anxiety, and heart palpitations. This medication may also cause your skin to be more sensitive to sunlight than it is normally. Exposure to sunlight, even for brief periods of time, may cause a skin rash, itching, redness or other discoloration of the skin, or a severe sunburn.

One of the little twists that makes treating FMS challenging is the fact that the side effects of the medications usually kick in right away,

---

Dealing with Dry Mouth

Tricyclic antidepressants may cause mouth dryness. For temporary relief, use sugarless gum or candy, melt bits of ice in your mouth, or use a saliva substitute. However, if your mouth continues to feel dry for more than 2 weeks, check with your doctor or dentist. Continuing dryness of the mouth may increase the chance of dental disease, including tooth decay, gum disease, and fungus infections.[20]

while the desired benefits may not be noticeable for 2 to 3 weeks. But if you can hold out, you'll find the side effects diminishing when the benefits take over.

If you do not want to deal with the side effects of tricyclic antidepressants or if you receive no symptom relief after several weeks, do not stop taking this medicine without first checking with your doctor. He or she may want you to reduce the amount you are using gradually before stopping completely. This may help prevent a possible worsening of your condition and reduce the possibility of withdrawal symptoms such as headache, nausea, and an overall feeling of discomfort.[21]

Selective Serotonin Reuptake Inhibitors

Selective serotonin reuptake inhibitors (SSRIs) is a very clear and descriptive name for this group of antidepressant medications. If you read these words from right to left, you'll have a good idea of how they work. SSRIs inhibit (or slow down) the reuptake (or the reabsorption) of serotonin, a brain neurotransmitter. This is done selectively without disrupting the function of other neurotransmitters and causing unwanted side effects (as sometimes happens with tricyclic antidepressants). Because SSRIs work by increasing the activity of the chemical serotonin in the brain, they are often used to treat FMS.

> *B*ecause SSRIs work by increasing the activity of the chemical serotonin in the brain, they are often used to treat FMS.

Some SSRIs commonly used to treat FMS are fluoxetine (Prozac), paroxetine (Paxil), sertraline (Zoloft), and citalopram (Celexa). These medicines are available only with your doctor's prescription.

Praise for SSRIs in the treatment of FMS is mixed. A study of 40 FMS patients between the ages of 18 and 65 compared the effectiveness and side effects of the tricyclic antidepressant amitriptyline with the SSRI sertraline. This study demonstrated that both were equally effective in measures evaluating pain, quality of sleep, fatigue, swelling, stiffness, numbness,

"Off-Label" Use

Once a medicine has been approved for marketing for a certain use, experience may show that it is also useful for other medical problems. Although these uses are not included in product labeling, tricyclic antidepressants are used in certain patients with the following "off-label" medical conditions: attention deficit hyperactivity disorder, bulimia, cocaine withdrawal, headache prevention, itching with hives due to cold temperature exposure, narcolepsy, neurogenic pain, panic disorder, stomach ulcer, and urinary incontinence.[22]

and number of tender points. However, sertraline had less reported side effects.[23] On the other hand, three studies of fluoxetine showed improvement in depression and sleep disturbance, but no effect on relief of pain at tender points was found.[24] For this reason, Dr. Robert Bennett recommends Zoloft, Paxil, and Prozac only for the 30 percent of FMS patients who also have depression.[25]

Because these drugs tend to interfere with sleep, they are often taken in the morning to fight daily fatigue and increase alertness, while a more sedating medication (such as a tricyclic antidepressant) is taken at night.

Precautions While Using SSRIs

Side effects of SSRIs include insomnia, dry mouth, headache, nausea, and diarrhea. On the upside, SSRIs do not cause the weight gain associated with tricyclics, but on the down side, you may lose your sex drive.

You should avoid drinking alcoholic beverages while taking this medication and make sure you know how you react to any SSRI before you drive, use machines, or do anything else that could be dangerous if you are not alert or well coordinated.

Do not take any SSRI within 2 weeks of taking a monoamine oxidase (MAO) inhibitor (furazolidone, phenelzine, procarbazine, selegiline, or tranylcypromine), and do not take an MAO inhibitor for at least 5 weeks after taking this medication. If you do, you may develop extremely high blood pressure or convulsions.

> *Do not take any SSRI within 2 weeks of taking a monoamine oxidase (MAO) inhibitor, and do not take an MAO inhibitor for at least 5 weeks after taking this medication.*

Do not stop taking this medicine without first checking with your doctor. He or she may want you to reduce gradually the amount you are taking before stopping completely. This is to decrease the chance of having discontinuation symptoms such as agitation, anxiety, dizziness, feeling of constant movement of self or surroundings, headache, increased sweating, nausea, trembling or shaking, trouble sleeping or walking, or unusual tiredness.[26]

Antidepressants in Action

Tricyclic antidepressants and SSRIs have changed the life of Karen, a 34-year-old partner in a public relations firm. When she was in college, Karen began to feel stiff and achy. "I thought maybe it was because I had stopped swimming competitively and my body was kind of adjusting to not being so athletic," she remembers. For about 5 years after college graduation, the pain increased, especially in her back. When the pain became unbearable, Karen went to her primary care doctor, who ordered x rays and MRIs, which found nothing significant. He also ordered blood tests, which showed an elevated Rh level. Without much else to offer, he prescribed 600 milligrams of Daypro, an anti-inflammatory medication, to be taken twice a day, and he suggested physical therapy. The therapist recommended an elastic back brace from her ribs to hips. Unfortunately, none of this gave Karen pain relief. "The medication and physical therapy did nothing for the total body pain—and it didn't even help my back," she says.

The pains and exhaustion continued, and Karen's primary care doctor sent her to a rheumatologist, who diagnosed fibromyalgia and told her to continue taking the anti-inflammatory medication and to consider pain management therapy. "I was glad to finally understand what was causing all my pain," says Karen, "and to know that it wasn't all in my head, but I wasn't very happy with the treatment. I don't like taking medications, and I wanted to become pregnant, so it really bothered me to be taking drugs that I knew had side effects and that weren't helping me anyway." Because the medication wasn't working, Karen stopped taking it and decided to just deal with the pain "naturally" as best she could.

Surprisingly, Karen did find pain relief in pregnancy. "The whole time I was pregnant and for about a year afterward I really felt much better," she recalls. "I thought that whatever it was that caused my pain was going away." But then the pains and exhaustion started again, and for the following 2 years she suffered through good days and bad days—alternating among Aleve, Motrin, and Tylenol. (Spending an hour and a half commuting every day to work didn't help!)

Recently the pain increased dramatically, and Karen changed doctors. "The first rheumatologist seemed to have the attitude I should just take these anti-inflammatories and learn to live with the pain. But the first thing my new doctor did was to explain that the anti-inflammatories won't stop the pain of fibromyalgia. Instead, after spending a lot of time talking to me about fibromyalgia, he prescribed antidepressants."

At first Karen was surprised and concerned by this treatment. "I was afraid he thought I was depressed and that the pain was all mental," she remembers. But her doctor explained that for some people with FMS, taking antidepressants at dosages much lower than would be prescribed for people with depression reduces the pain. Karen left with prescriptions for 20 milligrams of Paxil (an SSRI) to be taken in the morning and 20 milligrams of Pamelor (a tricyclic antidepressant) to be taken at night to improve her sleep.

> *For some people with FMS, taking antidepressants at dosages much lower than would be prescribed for people with depression reduces the pain.*

"It took 2 months to work, but then I noticed an absolutely tremendous change," says Karen with a wide smile. "I used to hurt so much that I'd wake up feeling like I got hit by a car. It was so painful to walk to the bathroom; I felt like I was 90 years old. And during the day, even though I'd push myself and do everything I had to do, I felt so exhausted. But now I have so much more energy because I can sleep, and the pain reduction is unbelievable. I have a little bit of a dry mouth and dry eyes because of the medication, but my doctor says these low dosages are safe for long-term use, so although I never thought I'd be taking pills every day of my life, I wouldn't give them up now for anything. This has changed my whole life."

Karen admits that she is also supposed to be doing 30 minutes of aerobic exercise every day and hasn't been able to find the time away from her job and her 4-year-old, but she knows that's one more thing she might do in the future to further help herself live with fibromyalgia.

Muscle Relaxants

Prescription muscle relaxants such as cyclobenzaprine (Flexeril), carisoprodol (Soma), dantrolene (Dantrium), zanaflex (Tizanidine), and baclofen (Lioresal) act on the central nervous system to treat muscle pain and tightness. For some people, these medications can relieve the spasms, cramping, and tightness of muscles common in FMS.

Although exactly how muscle relaxants work on the symptoms of FMS is not known, it is thought that the pain relief is a byproduct of improved sleep. A sleep study by John Reynolds, M.D., and Harvey Moldofsky, M.D., found that muscle relaxants increased total sleep time and slightly decreased evening fatigue.[27] Unfortunately, muscle relaxants do not cure the muscle pains of FMS, but when used along with physical therapy, they can extend the time before the muscles cramp up again.

If you are using a muscle relaxant and going to physical therapy, be sure to tell your therapist. Dr. Vincent Sferra, a chiropractic physi-

Commonly Used Drug Treatment Options

Pain
Nonsteroidal anti-inflammatory drugs (ibuprofen, Celebrex)
Analgesics (Ultram)
Muscle relaxants (Flexeril, Soma, Dantrium, Tizanidine, Lioresal)
Narcotic analgesics (MS-Contin, OxyContin, methodone, Viodin, Percodan, morphine)
Trigger point injections of an anesthetic or low-dose cortisone

Sleep
Tricyclic antidepressants (Elavil, Sinequan, Pamelor)
Short-acting sleeping pills (Ambien, Sonata)

Fatigue
Selective serotonin reuptake inhibitors (SSRIs) (Prozac, Paxil, Zoloft, Celexa)

cian who is the director of Natural Medicine and Rehabilitation in Bridgewater, New Jersey, tries to wean his patients off muscle relaxants because he feels they can be counterproductive in this situation. "A systemic muscle relaxant relaxes a lot of things besides the tense muscles," he says. "You may have many weak muscles that do not need relaxing but rather need conditioning. Muscle relaxants can slow your progress."

Precautions While Using Muscle Relaxants

Muscle relaxants may cause dizziness, vision problems, confusion, constipation, dry mouth, light-headedness, nausea, unusual weakness (especially muscle weakness), clumsiness, or unsteadiness in some people.

Muscle relaxants that work on the central nervous system (e.g., Soma, Lioresal, and Flexeril) have sedating properties that can cause daytime drowsiness and often limit their use to nighttime hours. The muscle relaxants that work peripherally on the muscles (e.g., Dantrium) are much less sedating. Diabetics should know that this medicine may cause blood sugar levels to rise. If you notice a change in the results of your blood or urine sugar test or if you have any questions about this, check with your doctor.

> *Muscle relaxants do not cure the muscle pains of FMS, but when used along with physical therapy, they can extend the time before the muscles cramp up again.*

Unwanted effects may also occur if the medicine is stopped suddenly. Do not abruptly stop taking this medicine. Check with your doctor for the best way to reduce gradually the amount you are taking before stopping completely.[28]

Sleeping Pills

Because your sleep is so often disturbed and nonrestful, you may take a sleeping pill to get through the night—but be cautious. *Sleeping pill* is a very broad term used to refer to any chemical agent that produces drowsiness. Each works by depressing the central nervous system in some manner, and some do this in ways that are ineffective and even counterproductive in the treatment of FMS. Dr. Giuffre explains that sedative sleeping pill medications (such as barbiturates, benzodiazepines, and over-the-counter products such as Sominex, Nytol, and Compoze) distort the normal sleep patterns by reducing the time spent in deep sleep (stages 3 and 4) and increasing time spent in shallow sleep (stages 1 and 2), causing more periods of wakefulness during the night. "This is especially disruptive for people with fibromyalgia," explains Dr. Giuffre, "because they already have trouble spending adequate time in the deep sleep stages where important restorative hormones are released, and they already are troubled by frequent awakenings from the lighter sleep stages by their pain and discomfort. Taking the wrong sleeping pill will compound these problems."

The "right" sleeping pill can be hard to find, but with a little trial-and-error sampling and lots of patience, you might find any of the following medications that are commonly prescribed for the sleep problems of fibromyalgia to be helpful:

- **Tricyclic antidepressants.** As already explained in detail, tricyclic antidepressants taken in doses much lower than those prescribed to treat depression can be very effective "sleeping pills."

- **Muscle relaxants.** Some muscle relaxants (such as carisoprodol [Soma]) are highly sedating. The effect lasts for about 6 hours.

> *D*iabetics should know that muscle relaxants may cause blood sugar levels to rise.

- **Short-acting sleep medications.** Some drugs marketed for insomnia (such as zolpidem [Ambien] and zaleplon [Sonata]) can increase evening sleepiness and daytime energy. Because they are short-acting (working for approximately 4 to 6 hours), the challenge is to find the right time to take them. Taken too soon in the evening, their effect will wear off between 2 and 4 o'clock in the morning when it is too late to take more without risking daytime sleepiness. If taken too late in the evening, there is the risk of daytime drowsiness. Due to the fear that these drugs may be habit forming, some physicians recommend that they be reserved for times of pain flares and exceptionally disrupted sleep.

Harvey Moldofsky, M.D., of the University of Toronto, tested 16 people with fibromyalgia who took 10 milligrams per night of zolpidem (Ambien). He found that the drug decreased the amount of time it took these people to fall asleep, decreased nighttime awakenings, increased daytime energy, and increased evening sleepiness.[29]

Many people with fibromyalgia also suffer limb movement disorders such as restless legs syndrome (RLS) and periodic limb movements (PLMs) during sleep. These disorders make it very difficult to sleep peacefully because they cause the arms and legs to jerk involuntarily and can create the need to move the legs constantly to find relief. These sleep disorders are believed to be caused by a lack of the brain neurotransmitter dopamine. Medications that raise dopamine levels or mimic the brain chemical may successfully ease this sleep problem. Commonly used drugs include levodopa/caribidopa (Sinemet) and bromocriptine (Parlodel).

Narcotic Analgesics

Narcotic analgesics such as MS-Contin, OxyContin, methodone, Vicodin, Percodan, and morphine are often used to relieve intense, acute pain and cancer pain, but their use in the treatment of FMS is a controversial topic. The Arthritis Foundation pamphlet on FMS says that narcotics are "ineffective and should be avoided because of their potential side effects."[30] A recent *Bulletin of Rheumatic Diseases* states that "narcotic analgesics have little or no place in the management of FMS."[31] Yet the American Pain Society, the American Academy for Pain Medicine, and the Federation of State Medical Boards have endorsed guidelines for the safe use of opioids in the management of chronic pain disorders.[32] So what can you believe?

Many physicians and researchers offering hope to people with FMS in uncontrolled pain believe that although no studies have been completed on the use of narcotics in the treatment of FMS, there's no reason to believe that the pain of FMS cannot be improved by narcotics. This is the opinion of well-known researcher and patient advocate Robert Bennett, M.D., of Oregon Health Sciences University in Portland, Oregon. "It's my experience," he says, "that in certain circumstances and with a clear understanding of what narcotics can and can't do, there are some patients with fibromyalgia who are helped by this kind of medical treatment."

The decision to use narcotics, however, is never an easy one. Dr. Bennett believes the decision is really up to the person in pain. "As a doctor, I have to be honest and admit that I can't tell how much pain a person is in. It's partly up to the patient to decide in what circumstance narcotics might be used. If a person has pain that is not being controlled by other means, if we've tried other medications, if I've known this person for a long time and feel she is emotionally stable and she has not had addiction problems in the past with alcohol or any other substance, and if she tells me that the pain is unbearable, she should have the choice of trying narcotic medications."

But before writing the prescription, Dr. Bennett makes sure his patients have realistic expectations and know the unwanted side effects they may experience. "It's important before going on narcotics that the patient understands that these drugs are not going to cure the pain," he notes. "They will reduce the pain by about 50 percent and may make people more functional, but they will not give a complete cure. They often cause side effects such as mental confusion, constipation, nausea, and itching. Some people may become addicted to them (about 5 percent of users)."

According to Dr. Bennett, this question of addiction needs some clarification. "Addiction is the same as substance abuse," he explains. "It is using a drug for nontherapeutic purposes. It is the state in which people exhibit antisocial behavior and lie and cheat and steal to get the drug. Very, very few people become addicted when prescribed narcotics under closely supervised medical care."

Elliott Gardner, Ph.D., agrees. Speaking at the 1999 American Pain Society meeting, he stated, "The vast majority of human beings do not have the genetic proclivity to use drugs. If you give these individuals opioids for whatever reason, such as relief of pain, they will not lapse into drug-taking addictive patterns because they don't have the genetic proclivity. On the best evidence to date, somewhere around 5 percent of the human population has this genetic proclivity—so the vast majority of patients are not going to be turned into

addicts simply because they have been administered opioids for prolonged periods of time, even at very high doses."[33]

On the other hand, dependency and tolerance—states often confused with addiction—are to be expected with long-term use of many
drugs. *Dependency* means that once you start tak-
ing a drug, you can't suddenly stop without getting a withdrawal reaction. "All this means," says
Dr. Bennett, "is that you have to wean off of them
slowly. Tolerance means that over time you may
need an increased dosage to produce the same effect. Fortunately, when this happens the side effects do not increase; in fact, they often decrease."
Dr. Bennett emphasizes, "Dependence and tolerance are not the same as addiction."

So why are doctors so reluctant to prescribe
narcotics for people with FMS who have uncon-
trolled pain? Dr. Bennett believes it is because doctors on the whole
are very poorly educated on the use of narcotics and prefer to avoid
the bother:

> **Addiction?**
>
> In the past 20 years I've only had 2 patients out of about 100 on narcotics who became addicted. Yet many doctors deny narcotic treatment because they confuse dependence with addiction.
>
> —ROBERT BENNETT, M.D.

> Doctors can't play around with these patients if they prescribe nar-
> cotics. They have to see them on a regular basis and take time to ed-
> ucate them about dependency. There is a lot of FDA-required record
> keeping, and doctors fear the scrutiny of medical review boards. It is
> a big hassle for doctors to give these out on a regular basis, and they
> don't like doing that.
>
> I don't use narcotics a lot. Only about 10 percent of my FMS pa-
> tients take them, but if they are helping a person function more fully,
> they should be given and continued. Patients who find relief from
> narcotics and can bear the side effects can stay on them indefinitely.
> They will experience tolerance, and the dosage will need to be in-
> creased. Many doctors consider these patients to be "drug seeking"
> and may contribute to the syndrome known as "pseudoaddictions" by
> adopting pejorative attitudes and denying increases in dosage.

The Morphine Patch

To sidestep the digestive problems associated with narcotics, some doctors prescribe transdermal patches that are placed on the skin to release the medication directly into the blood system. The fentanyl patch (Duragesic) releases high doses of morphine to treat chronic pain in this manner. Low-dose versions are being tested.

Precautions While Using Narcotics for Pain

If you choose to give narcotics a try, keep the following information in mind. First, if you will be taking this medicine for a long time (such as for several months), your doctor should check your progress at regular visits.

Second, narcotic analgesics may cause some people to become drowsy, dizzy, or light-headed or to feel a false sense of well-being. Make sure you know how you react to this medicine before you drive, use machines, or do anything else that could be dangerous if you are dizzy or are not alert and clearheaded .

Third, nausea or vomiting may occur, especially after the first couple of doses. This effect may go away if you lie down for a while. However, if nausea or vomiting continues, check with your medical doctor.

Finally, if you have been taking this medicine regularly for several weeks or more, do not suddenly stop using it without first checking with your doctor. He or she may want you to reduce gradually the amount you are taking before stopping completely, in order to lessen the chance of withdrawal side effects.[34]

Trigger Point Injections

Many physicians will treat localized painful areas with injections of medications (such as the local anesthetic lidocaine) into the painful areas of the muscles. Also used are cortisone derivatives, such as prednisolone. This technique is most often applied in the treatment of the trigger points of the myofascial pain syndrome (MPS), which many people with FMS also have. In fact, roughly 65 percent of people with FMS have these painful trigger points.[35] As explained in chapter 2, these trigger points are areas of tight, knotted muscles that can be very painful, and when pressed send shooting pain to other areas of the body. An injection of an anesthetic (sometimes mixed with low-dose cortisone) can ease the pain. This treatment is most effective when followed immediately by a deep-tissue massage and in conjunction with at-home stretching exercises and physical or occupational therapy. The physician may repeat injections each week; treatment up to 3 weeks may be necessary for extremely troublesome areas.

Trigger point injection is most effective when followed immediately by a deep-tissue massage and in conjunction with at-home stretching exercises and physical or occupational therapy.

Although the trigger points of MPS often respond well to trigger point injections, it is not always practical to treat the tender points of FMS with these injections because they are so numerous throughout the body. But Dr. Yunus feels that if there are one to four extremely bothersome areas, trigger point injections may be a valuable adjunctive therapy. "The benefit of this treatment," he says, "lasts 2 to 4 months. I rarely inject a patient's tender points more frequently than every 2 to 3 months."

Combination Therapy

In many FMS cases, one medication alone is not enough to control the multiple symptoms. Your doctor may give you several prescriptions to work on different symptoms at different times of the day. For example, you may take Elavil to help you sleep at night, Paxil to give you energy during the day, and Ultram to battle pain. During a flare period, your doctor may increase the dosage of some medications or add additional ones.

In some instances, your doctor may combine medications to gain a synergistic bonus. Research has shown that combining doses of certain drugs may work better and have fewer side effects than either drug used alone. Don Goldenberg, M.D., chief of rheumatology at the Newton-Wellesley Hospital in Massachusetts, leads the way in this area of research. He has done a number of studies that explore the combined effects of drugs commonly used to treat fibromyalgia. A good example of how this works is found in his early work with FMS patients who took naproxen (found in Aleve) and amitriptyline (an antidepressant) twice daily. Trying these drugs separately and in combination to determine their effectiveness, he found that the patients taking the combination therapy did better than those taking just one of these therapies when reporting their level of pain.[36]

In a more recent study, Dr. Goldenberg examined the effect of the tricyclic antidepressant amitriptyline (Elavil and others) used in combination with the SSRI antidepressant fluoxetine (Prozac). Again, Dr. Goldenberg tested these drugs alone and in combination in 19 patients with fibromyalgia and found that both drugs given separately showed definite improvement in muscle pain, sleep disturbances, and daily functioning. What was most interesting was his discovery that the two medications together did better than either one individually with less side effects. Amitriptyline can cause grogginess or fatigue, while fluoxetine tends to make people feel more awake and cheerful. Giving fluoxetine in the morning and amitriptyline in the evening resulted in few side effects. Dr. Goldenberg estimates that a combination of fluoxetine and amitriptyline could help about half of all people with fibromyalgia.[37]

Dr. Goldenberg estimates that a combination of fluoxetine and amitriptyline could help about half of all people with fibromyalgia.

Dr. Goldenberg believes combination therapy may be more effective in treating the symptoms of fibromyalgia than a single drug because different medications affect neurotransmitters like serotonin differently and create a synergistic effect when taken together. "There are far too many possible combinations of analgesics, antidepressants, anti-inflammatories, and antianxiety drugs to state right now which combination will work best for all people with FMS," says Dr. Goldenberg, "but when single drug therapies are not working, combination therapy is an approach your physician might try."

Benzodiazepines, corticosteroids, melatonin, and NSAIDs are no better than placebo and may be associated with significant side effects. Therefore, they have no role in the routine management of FMS.[38]

USE WITH CAUTION

Many of the medications that are used to treat the symptoms of FMS, such as Ultram, tricyclic antidepressants, SSRIs, muscle relaxants, and narcotics, can cause tolerance or dependence. If you take any medications for a long period of time, talk to your doctor if you notice that you are not receiving the same benefits you previously had at the same dosage. This may be a sign of tolerance, and you may have to have the dosage adjusted or you may need to switch to a different medication. Also talk to your doctor if you feel you need the medication to function and begin to feel very anxious at the thought of running out of pills (a possible indication of dependence or even addiction).

You also need to be aware that these drugs can cause dangerous interactions with other central nervous system depressants. Some examples of CNS depressants are alcohol; antihistamines or medicine for hay fever, other allergies, or colds; sedatives, tranquilizers, or sleeping medicine; prescription pain medicine or narcotics; barbiturates; medicine for seizures; muscle relaxants; or anesthetics, including some dental anesthetics. Be sure to check with your medical doctor before taking any of these medications while you are on a CNS depressant for the treatment of fibromyalgia.

This is often easy to say, but not so easy to do consistently. It's understandable that if you take medications daily, after a while you may forget how potent they can be and how careful you have to be about interactions. This is what makes Kim worry about her sister Janet. Kim's 57-year-old sister, Janet, has fibromyalgia, and although Kim understands the disease and knows how debilitating it can be, she worries about the medications her sister lives on. "The pain started as migraine headaches when Janet was a teenager," Kim remembers. "She was on the Darvon [a narcotic analgesic] until she was about 40 years old, and during those years she became addicted to it. She also developed degenerative disc problems in her back, as well as osteoporosis, that also created a chronic pain situation. Doctors put Janet on Soma [a muscle relaxant] along with antidepressants, along with goodness knows what else."

Ten years ago, Janet admitted herself to an inpatient program for drug addiction, but she left abruptly. "I don't think that people who are addicted to prescription drugs see themselves as addicts," says Kim. "My sister says that all she's trying to do is control her pain, and she can't give up the medication if she wants to function. And I'm sure she figures that since the pills are prescribed by her doctor, why should she have to give them up? I don't know if my sister is the type of patient who hops around from doctor to doctor until she gets what she wants, but I don't think so. I do think she has an addictive personality and that she is the kind of person who has blind faith in her doctor and does what's she's told without asking questions. That makes me very concerned.

"Of course, if she's addicted to something that she can't function without, I can't be her judge and jury on that; I might choose the drug over the pain myself if I were in her place. But I do worry about the effects of these drugs on her kidneys. I also worry about drug interactions that I have seen, and I worry about the fact that she does have an occasional glass of wine—I've seen her become noticeably impaired after only one sip. I'm afraid she'll get behind the wheel of a car thinking she's just fine because she's had only one drink. I just wish there was one person who was keeping track of all the different pills she's taking and could help her understand the dangers of mixing the pills she lives on every day with even a sip of alcohol."

Kim's concerns are very real and valid. If you are taking medications to manage your fibromyalgia as well as other medical conditions, make sure that your primary care doctor or a central pharmacist is keeping track of possible drug interactions. Also be very careful about any over-the-counter medications you may take for something as simple as a cold.

TRIAL AND ERROR

You should feel hopeful knowing that doctors and medical researchers now have many drugs that have been proven to help relieve the symptoms of fibromyalgia. But don't expect any of these medications to be a complete cure or to work flawlessly. Because the symptoms of FMS vary from one person to another, because many medications that work well for one person do nothing for another, and because the side effects of some of these medications can be worse than the illness, it may take time and patience to find the medications just right for you. Remember, there are no drugs formulated and labeled specifically for the treatment of fibromyalgia, so you and your doctor have to figure out which ones of the many possibilities will be best.

Remember, there are no drugs formulated and labeled specifically for the treatment of fibromyalgia, so you and your doctor have to figure out which ones of the many possibilities will be best.

Finding relief may require taking a number of pills. Some people take medication for pain and fatigue in the morning and other medications for sleep disturbances at night. Some start on a low dosage of particular medications and need to increase the dosage until they feel relief. Some need to try different medications until they find one that works.

Speaking Out

Take a look at what people with fibromyalgia said about their medication on an online bulletin board:

- "My primary doctor had me on naproxen and then switched me to Vioxx. Both made me sick and didn't help. Now I'm on Sinequan and I feel much better."

- "I started out on Paxil and it made me sick to my stomach. Now I'm on Prozac and doing fine."

- "I was switched to Celexa, first on 20 milligrams, and then onto 40 milligrams. They also increased my trazodone up to 50 milligrams. Tomorrow I start on Effexor."

- "I started low doses of Neruontin, and it didn't help with the burning pain. It was increased to 2,400 milligrams a day and that really helped stop the burning pain. Now the doc has me up to 3,200 milligrams because my life is extremely stressful, which makes FMS more painful."

- "I take Trazodone, 100 milligrams at night for sleep, along with 10 milligrams Flexeril. (I sleep very well now.) I also take other meds like Paxil, Tylenol with Codeine, and Xanax."

You may be lucky and find a helpful regimen right away, but if not, don't hesitate to keep asking for changes in your medication. If you have given a prescribed medicine a month of your time (and some do take this long to work effectively) and see no change in your condition, speak up! Many patients with fibromyalgia worry that they seem to be nagging their doctors with so many aches and pains and problems that they don't want to "bother" them with another request for new medicine, but that's how this syndrome is managed.

TREATING OTHER CONDITIONS THAT ACCOMPANY FIBROMYALGIA

Treatment for fibromyalgia is distinct and separate from the treatment for the other medical conditions that you may have along with FMS. If you have irritable bowel syndrome, for example, your doctor may give you an antispasmodic drug to ease the cramping pain. If you have hypertension, you may take a beta-blocker like atenolol. If you have urinary infections, you may take an antibiotic. Do not sacrifice your medical needs in another area because you're sensitive to the time and effort your doctor puts into finding the right treatment for FMS. Remember, the health of your body is a priority, and you are your only advocate. Speak up when you need care.

Do not sacrifice your medical needs in another area because you're sensitive to the time and effort your doctor puts into finding the right treatment for FMS.

When you find yourself taking various medications to treat a number of different medical problems, be cautious, and make sure one central person is keeping track of all the medications. This may be your primary care doctor or even your pharmacist, but someone must be aware of each medication you are taking to ensure that there is no danger of drug interactions among them. One drug can negate the benefits of another; some drugs can react with others to cause dangerous side effects; some drugs simply will not work as expected when used in combination with other drugs. To get the most out of your medications, make sure there is someone watching for possible drug interactions.

SEARCHING FOR RELIEF

Although there is no cure for fibromyalgia, there is hope for symptom relief and normal functioning—if you are persistent and determined to find something that works for you. Unfortunately, too many people with fibromyalgia needlessly suffer day after day on treatment regimens that just aren't working. Fifty-year-old Raylene is one of them.

Raylene first started having pain problems in her back in 1982. "After tests showed nothing was wrong, my doctor assumed that because I was female my pain must have been caused by depression. He said that my problems with sleep were a sign of depression and the aches and pains were because I wasn't sleeping. So without any major concern, I was given the antidepressant amitriptyline. Because, ironically, this medication is often prescribed for people who have fibromyalgia, I did start to feel better and started to assume the doctor was right about my symptoms being caused by depression." However, as Raylene's spirits would rise, she would stop taking the medication, and her pain level would go way up again.

> *Too many people with fibromyalgia needlessly suffer day after day on treatment regimens that just aren't working.*

Later, in 1984, Raylene began to suspect that something still wasn't right. At this time she was going to a university. ("I got started late in life," she says.) One day she found herself on the second-floor landing looking up to the third floor where her math class was held, and she realized that because she was so sore and exhausted, there was no way she could get her legs to go any farther. "By this time I was sure something was very wrong with me. I knew this just couldn't be normal."

Then, after she graduated from the university in 1988, Raylene got a teaching job and struggled through every day. Someone who was always on the go and who loved being very busy and never felt tired had turned into someone who taught school, went home, and went to bed every day, year after year.

During this time, Raylene was also in and out of the hospital for muscle spasms in her back and legs. "One time it happened in April while I was teaching; I just couldn't move. They called the ambulance, and I was taken out on a stretcher. The pain was so bad, I didn't go back to school for the rest of that school year." At that time, Raylene was diagnosed with "extreme stress" and given muscle relaxants and tranquilizers. This seemed bizarre to her because at this time in her life she was finally stress-free. She had a good job she liked, a steady paycheck, and no bills to worry about. But she was in pain, and no one could find any other explanation.

This went on and on until finally, in 1995, a neurologist diagnosed fibromyalgia. With a name for her pain, Raylene thought this was good news and maybe there was some relief in sight, but unfortunately her doctor believed fibromyalgia was a psychiatric condition. Willing to try anything to function better, Raylene went to a psychiatrist, feeling that if she needed psychological therapy, that would be fine with her as long as the pain and fatigue stopped. After one short meeting, the psychiatrist said, "You don't need to come back to me. Your problem is not stress related, and it's not in your head." Oddly enough, Raylene broke down and cried. "If this doctor had said that the pain was all in my head," says Raylene, "I figured it was something I could face and beat. That was my last hope." Discouraged, she felt that no one could help her.

At this time, Raylene's local doctor has put her on low-dose antidepressants for arthritis. "If I don't take these medications," she says, "I can't even get out of the house. If I do take them, I'm able to drag myself to school, and I mean *drag*. I'm having a hard, hard time. My life consists of standing on my feet all day, teaching 6- and 7-year-olds. During the day I have trouble focusing; I have a hard time remembering things, and it takes all I have to be patient with my students. Then I go home, have dinner, and fall into bed for the night by six o'clock. Every day, that's all I have the energy to do."

> *A*ll the fibromyalgia experts agree that medication alone cannot control the symptoms of fibromyalgia.

Sadly, Raylene's case shows very clearly that relief from the pain, fatigue, and sleep problems of fibromyalgia is not easy to come by. Unfortunately for her, it appears that her physician is not willing to put in the time and effort for the trial-and-error treatment process that FMS often requires.

Don't let this happen to you. Do not be afraid to try different types of medications, different doses, and different combinations until you find relief. And don't stop there. All the fibromyalgia experts agree that medication alone cannot control the symptoms of fibromyalgia. Dr. Joseph E. Scherger says, "There is no external magic bullet for FMS. People who walk into their doctor's office and say, 'Take it away,' have a false understanding of the nature of the problem. The person herself has to make the changes that are necessary to relieve the symptoms."

The good news is that virtually everyone can do this. The following chapters will give you more treatment strategies to help you take control of your life and gain improved health and function.

CHAPTER 4

Exercise and Relaxation Techniques

AFTER YOUR DOCTOR has prescribed whatever medications you both feel will help you function better, it's time to add exercise and relaxation techniques to your treatment regimen. Sorry, but these two pieces of your treatment plan cannot go on your long list of "things I don't have time for" or "things that only make me feel worse." Exercise and relaxation techniques that are carefully tailored to your needs and capabilities are absolutely vital to functioning well with fibromyalgia. But like so many other aspects of treating FMS, you must have patience and determination to find just the right person to guide you and just the right therapy programs to help your individual FMS circumstance.

This chapter will give you a few pointers to get you headed in the right direction, but this is the point in your treatment program where you have to take charge and decide what's best for you and what you want to do to help yourself. How often you get up and exercise or sit down and relax will be up to you—but many doctors, researchers, and people with fibromyalgia agree that exercise and relaxation are tools that can empower you to do something yourself to improve the way you feel.

Ken Giuffre, M.D., president of Trilobot Institute for Applied Cognitive Research in New Jersey, says, "No one is a helpless victim of pain. We all have the ability to do something about the way we perceive pain and directly affect the role pain plays in our lives. Physical exercise and relaxation therapies are two of the most commonly used lifestyle choices people make to take control of their pain."

> *E*xercise and relaxation techniques that are carefully tailored to your needs and capabilities are absolutely vital to functioning well with fibromyalgia.

Research supports the benefits of this choice. A study published in *Arthritis Care Research* on the value of relaxation training and exercise in the treatment of fibromyalgia reported excellent results. Those patients using relaxation or exercise as treatment therapies produced greater improvements in self-efficacy for function and a greater reduction of tender point pain as compared to the control group. (Control-group members who used neither relaxation nor exercise actually showed deterioration in tender point pain symptoms during this period.) The group that used both relaxation and exercise therapies best maintained benefits across a 2-year period.[1] This is just one study of many that confirms the value of exercise and relaxation in a comprehensive treatment program for FMS.

In this chapter you'll first take a look at what happens in your body when you exercise that eases the pain and fatigue of FMS, and then you'll find out how to determine the type, frequency, and intensity of exercise that is best for you. Then you'll explore the role of relaxation in the treatment of fibromyalgia and look at specific techniques that you can use starting today to put a stop to the stress response that is fueling your fatigue and pain.

GET UP AND GET MOVING

What's the last thing you want to do when you hurt all over and feel like you can't drag one foot in front of the other one more time? Of course, the answer is "exercise." Simple logic keeps telling you that daily exercise can't be good for fibromyalgia. When you're tired, you should rest—right? When you're in pain, you should take it easy—right? Everything you've ever learned about treating fatigue and pain tells you to stay away from exercise. But you also know that if you give into the temptation to rationalize your way out of exercising, you'll hurt even more and feel even more tired in the future. Aside from all the physical and psychological benefits of exercise, just doing it keeps you out of the vicious pain-exercise cycle. This is the cycle that begins when you say your muscles hurt too much to exercise; so you don't exercise and your muscles become unconditioned; then because your muscles are uncon-

> ### In Control
> Physical exercise and relaxation therapies are two of the most commonly used lifestyle choices people make to take control of their pain.
>
> —*KEN GIUFFRE, M.D.*

ditioned, they hurt even more and then you feel more strongly that you can't exercise; so you don't and the muscles become further unconditioned, and they hurt even more; and on and on and on (see figure 4.1).

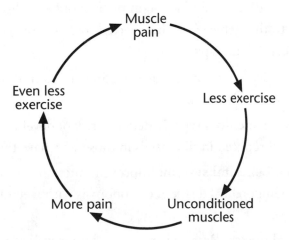

Figure 4.1—*Pain-Exercise Cycle*

Besides the value of using physical activity to keep you out of this pain cycle, other benefits of exercise in the management of chronic pain are measurable and physical:

- Regular moderate exercise releases brain chemicals such as adrenaline, serotonin, and norepinephrine that will boost our mood and relieve the pain-enhancing states of tension and depression.

- Exercise produces better sleep—a real benefit for anyone with FMS. Sound sleep allows the body the restorative time it needs to repair and rejuvenate.

- Exercise is a proven preventative medicine. It can prevent predisposition to painful arthritis, bone degeneration, and obesity that afflict many with FMS and compound the difficulty of treating this syndrome.

The overall positive effect of physical activity on health is underscored by published recommendations from the Centers for Disease Control and Prevention that highlight the benefits of regular exercise in the general population:

- **Cardiac disease.** Reduction in the risk of heart disease comparable to that achieved with hypertension control and estrogen replacement therapy.

- **Stroke.** Risk of stroke reduced by 50 percent in those who exercise regularly for years.

- **Diabetes mellitus type 2.** Reduced risk of developing the disease and reduced insulin needs in those who have the disease.

- **Musculoskeletal system:** Improved function and sense of well-being; reduced risk of osteoporosis with weight-bearing exercise.

- **Mental health:** Reduced anxiety and improved sense of well-being; improvement of minor depression.

- **Obesity:** Useful adjunct to reduction of caloric intake for slow, steady weight loss.

- **Preservation of function:** Gains in strength and function, even when exercise is started later in life.[2]

Physical medicine and rehabilitation specialist Douglas Ashendorf, M.D., believes that some form of exercise is necessary and essential in the treatment of fibromyalgia, regardless of other medications or interventions that may be used. "I consider medications, nerve blocks, and some surgeries to be adjuncts to an exercise program," he says. "Their purpose is to allow the patient to begin exercising earlier, more vigorously, and with less discomfort. I consider these modalities as 'tools in the toolbox'; however, a patient's rehabilitation success will ultimately depend on his or her lifetime dedication to exercise. That is the single and most important tool.

"But," warns Dr. Ashendorf, "trying to exercise away the pain without guidance and instruction from a person who understands fibromyalgia is often meaningless. A program that might include stretching, flexibility, strengthening, stabilization, retraining of movement or posture, and aerobics should be individualized for a patient by an experienced physical or occupational therapist. Finding the right program is a challenging task, but by no means an impossible one."

> *A patient's rehabilitation success will ultimately depend on his or her lifetime dedication to exercise. That is the single and most important tool.*
>
> —DOUGLAS ASHENDORF, M.D.

So if your doctor says, "I want you to exercise," ask for a prescription for physical therapy so that a trained professional can put you on the right track.

A Much Better Place

Kate's fibromyalgia developed as the result of a bad fall while mountain climbing 3 years ago when she was 49 years old. After about 8 hours of climbing, Kate slipped on her way back down and fell about 15 feet. Despite her pain, she finished the descent and went home to soak in a hot bath. Kate feels she never really recovered from this accident. Her lower right back kept signaling pain that eventually spread. "Soon pain was shooting from my hips down to my knees," Kate remembers. "My hips were searing; my back felt rigid; the pain was awful. It was a 3-year journey to figure out what was wrong. During that time when I didn't know what was going on, I tried everything to ease the pain. I tried yoga, meditation, stretching, acupuncture, hypnosis, swimming, physical therapy, and trigger point injections. You name it—I tried it. But nothing gave me relief. In fact, it was getting worse over time."

There were days during these years when Kate felt like she just couldn't get out of bed. She was suffering terrible fatigue and didn't want to have to walk across the room. "I went from doctor to doctor and tried all kinds of medication, and nothing worked. I know the doctors were all thinking I was a hypochondriac. I kept talking about pain, and they kept handing me narcotics. I can't tell you how many different medications I was on. I remember taking anti-inflammatories, Ultram, Daypro, trazodone—nothing helped. I just couldn't find relief."

Kate knows she probably could have handled her pain by staying drugged all day, but she had a business to run. "I own a marketing company, and I couldn't just let it go," says Kate. "Thank goodness for my husband. He picked up the slack in my darkest days; I don't know what I would have done without him." Then finally after 3 years of discouragement, Kate went to the Mayo Clinic. The intake doctor sent her to a specialist, who talked to her for awhile, did a tender point exam, and within minutes said, "You have fibromyalgia." Kate had never heard this word before. "It took me several days to learn how to pronounce it!"

Kate went home with a collection of stretching exercises, advice to get more rest, and a prescription for the antidepressant Serzone to improve the quality of her sleep. "What a downer," says Kate. "First I have to deal with an illness that I'm told is never going away, and then I'm trying to function on medication that made me feel like an absolute zombie. I found myself going back to bed at three o'clock in the afternoon." After about 3 weeks of this, Kate knew this wasn't the answer. She called the physical therapist who had been working with her before the diagnosis and knew her pain; she asked for some help or advice. He referred Kate to a rheumatologist who had fibromyalgia himself.

Her new doctor was, according to Kate, "a wonderful man." At their first meeting he spent 90 minutes with Kate, listening and talking to her. Then he prescribed three things:

1. Sleep and sleep deeply

2. Exercise every day

3. Reduce stress

"I looked at him like he was crazy," laughs Kate. "'I don't have time to exercise every day,' I thought. How in the world as a career professional could I find time to exercise every day? Reduce stress? My life is built around stress! But I took the advice, figuring, 'Why not? I've tried everything else.' And I can't begin to tell you how my life has turned around. For over a year I have exercised religiously, and I take half a tab (5 milligrams) of Flexeril [a muscle relaxant] and Ambien [a short-acting sleeping pill] to help me sleep deeply so my body can heal while I rest.

"The amazing part to me is that after 3 years of trying so many things, the answer to my problem has been so simple. I'm doing back exercises and aerobic exercises. I'm working hard, and the payoff is there. I'm not pain-free, but I'm a different woman. Whatever it was that caused my pain has eased. I never want to go back to feeling that kind of pain again. I know what my body is telling me, and I know the approach I'm using now is working for me. I'm in a much better place than I have been for a long, long time.

"I told my doctor that I really regretted that I couldn't get back on my treadmill. I used to really love my treadmill; it was like my best friend. He said, 'You can.' 'No,' I said. 'My back just won't support it. I can't.' He said, 'If you work into it, you can do it.' Well, I'm not going to say that I'm doing 45 minutes on my treadmill like I did before my accident, but I can use it for 10 minutes. I can do that, and that's a completely different place than where I was after the onset of fibromyalgia."

Jump-Starting an Exercise Program with Physical Therapy

Deciding that you will include exercise in your FMS management plan is a good first step toward feeling better. Then you need to take the second step—creating an exercise plan. If you exercise only occasionally, or too intensely, or incorrectly, you'll find your FMS symptoms getting worse, and you'll end up giving up exercise altogether.

> *If you exercise only occasionally, or too intensely, or incorrectly, you'll find your FMS symptoms getting worse, and you'll end up giving up exercise altogether.*

Mark Gostine, M.D., a nationally renowned fibromyalgia expert and cofounder of ProCare Systems (the nation's only medical management company specializing in the development of comprehensive pain programs), sees many people with chronic muscle or skeletal problems (such as FMS) who say they find no relief in exercising. "Probably the most common reasons for lack of pain relief," says Dr. Gostine, "is failure to exercise properly—either because the prescribed exercise is not tailored to the individual patient or because the patient does not persist in performing the exercise. If, for example, a person who cannot tolerate standing or walking for more than a few moments is made to exercise against resistance, the only result can be failure. No wonder the first comment from many of my patients is 'I hate exercise.'"

Most researchers who study FMS and exercise agree that you need support, encouragement, and supervision to get the most benefit out of this aspect of your treatment plan. If your doctor agrees that exercise would help you feel better, ask for a prescription for physical therapy (which should be covered under your health care insurance plan) from a therapist who is experienced with treating fibromyalgia.

Dr. Vincent Sferra, a chiropractic physician who is the director of Natural Medicine and Rehabilitation in Bridgewater, New Jersey, believes FMS is best treated with a holistic program that includes exercise, initially under the guidance of a physical therapist. He says there are three reasons that physical therapy is a good place to start.

First, exercise reconditions the muscles of the body. "I'd say that 80 to 100 percent of the people with fibromyalgia have muscles that need to be strengthened and conditioned." These deconditioned muscles use excess energy for a given task, which contributes to the feeling of extreme fatigue. These muscles may also be susceptible to microtraumas that are additionally aggravated because they do not benefit from the healing and restorative power of stage 4 sleep that people with FMS often do not have (as explained in chapter 3).

"I've seen many patients who come in and explain that they've been told by a medical specialist to remain passive and not 'hurt' their muscles," says Dr. Sferra. "But this attitude increases the likelihood that the symptoms of fibromyalgia will increase in intensity. The less you stimulate the nerve receptors for motion in all the muscles and joints of the body, the more prone you will be to feeling pain. But if you work to regularly stimulate those motion receptors through exercise, you help abort the messages of pain that constantly bombard the system. As difficult as it can be, it's very important to become involved in a program of reconditioning to offset some of the fatigue and joint pain that without action can make you bedridden."

There are many ways therapists can recondition your muscles:

- **Passive therapies** physically work the muscles and joints without your active involvement. This kind of exercise can recondition muscles in many ways; most notably, they may (1) move and lengthen muscles that have become too short and tight,

(2) mobilize faulty joint mechanics that may have become stiff due to deconditioning, and (3) reduce tension within the muscle fascia through manual manipulation of muscle and joint. Passive exercises may employ techniques such as massage, heat, therapeutic stretching, and electric stimulation.

- **Stabilization training** can also recondition muscles. This method teaches you how to activate some of the deeper muscles of the core so you can gain control of and stabilize muscles such as those in the pelvic, low-back, and shoulder areas. If a person is unable to endure reasonable muscle tension or to remain stable in the deeper muscles, exercise of any kind can be difficult.

- **Sensory motor training** teaches the nerves how to communicate better with the muscles and joints. The nerves need to know when the body is going into a vulnerable position so they can activate the muscles to react against injury. It's like when you slip off the curb and you catch yourself before spraining your ankle—your nervous system sent a quick message to the muscles to keep you from injury. But when the muscles are deconditioned and fatigued, you have less of an ability to have this kind of sensory motor response. Specific exercises can train the sensory motor response.

- **Overall body reconditioning** can begin after the body has been carefully stabilized. Physical therapists will prescribe safe and beneficial exercises, a combination of cardiovascular and cardiorespiratory training that includes a little bit each of strength, endurance, and flexibility training.

The second reason physical therapy is helpful to fibromyalgics is that exercise corrects muscular imbalances and postural faults that develop as the body tries to compensate for the pain of fibromyalgia as well as other overlapping conditions. Dr. Sferra says that those with depression or myofascial pain syndrome, for example, more than likely have imbalances that need physical therapy. "They may have joint dysfunction through the neck and shoulder blades and the lower back," he explains. "They need to strengthen these weak links, release tight muscles, and lengthen taut muscles. They may have the muscle knots of trigger points or adhesions and lesions on the muscle fascia that need to be worked on with manual and muscle-balancing techniques. At the same time, the muscles in pain due to fibromyalgia need to be handled with gentle release techniques."

> *Exercise corrects muscular imbalances and postural faults that develop as the body tries to compensate for the pain of fibromyalgia as well as other overlapping conditions.*

Finally, physical therapy gives you a structured and supervised program. Too many people are told by their physicians that they should exercise but are then sent off to figure out on their own how to exercise in a way that will help not hurt them. "I can't emphasize enough," says Dr. Sferra, "that a person who tries to do the right thing by exercising without guidance or by following a videotape made for healthy individuals without fibromyalgia will become very discouraged and give up when the exercise creates more pain and more problems. A physical therapy program gives you education, structure, and motivation. These three things will keep you working toward symptom relief much longer than you could do on your own. A physical therapist can explain what exercises are right for your individual needs, why certain exercises may hurt, and how this pain does not necessarily mean you are doing harm to your body. This gives you the confidence and reassurance you need to continue."

Not All Physical Therapy Programs Are Created Equal

Once you convince your doctor and your insurance company that you do need prescribed physical therapy, you'll need to spend some time finding a competent physical therapist. This is as important—and sometimes as difficult—as finding the "right" physician. Dr. Sferra offers these guidelines to help you identify the kind of therapist who can best work with the pain of fibromyalgia.

"You need a therapist," he says, "who has experience and training in the management of fibromyalgia pain. You need one who will create a program around your individual needs. You need a program that is different from the one created for the person who needs to strengthen a torn rotator cuff or rebuild muscle lost to atrophy while healing from a skiing accident. You may need a program that is different even from the one of the person sitting next to you who also has fibromyalgia. (Some people with FMS can do 3 minutes on a stationary bike right at the start; others can't even get themselves up on the bike.) You also need a therapist who understands the complexities of fibromyalgia and understands your pain and fatigue.

"Just as there are still uninformed and unsympathetic doctors out there," Dr. Sferra continues, "there are also physical therapists who do not understand your illness and will not believe that you really can't do what they ask you to do. You need someone who understands that physical therapy is a challenge for you and that you need support and encouragement."

Finding a Physical Therapist

When looking for a physical therapist, be sure to ask these questions:

- Do you work with people suffering chronic pain and fatigue?

- Do you work with people who have fibromyalgia?

- Do you have a therapy program that specifically addresses the pain of fibromyalgia?

- What is the basic outline of a typical program? (It should include at least aerobic exercise, stretching, muscle strengthening, correct posture, and proper body mechanics in carrying out daily tasks.)

How long will you need a structured physical therapy program? As with every aspect of treating FMS, the answer to this question is different for each person. Dr. Sferra feels that sometime within 3 to 6 months you should feel confident about helping yourself at home to recondition your body and correct muscular imbalances. But regardless of how long you use a supervised program, all FMS experts agree that the program of exercise rehabilitation must be continued at home. As Dr. Sferra says, "Physical therapy and exercise are not about curing fibromyalgia; they're about learning how to help yourself feel better and become stronger."

> *Regardless of how long you use a supervised program, all FMS experts agree that the program of exercise rehabilitation must be continued at home.*

Just What the Doctor Ordered

When Sue was diagnosed with fibromyalgia during her first year of marriage, her doctor put the 24-year-old on a simple treatment program that seemed to be just what she needed. "My doctor said that exercise, stretching, and getting enough sleep were the best things I could do for myself," remembers Sue, "and he was right."

The doctor gave Sue a prescription for Elavil (a tricyclic antidepressant) to help her sleep. And she began going to physical therapy three times a week to work out the muscle knots in her neck and shoulders that were painful and contributed to her headaches; lastly, he handed her a prescription for physical therapy three times a week.

"My physical therapist was very good," remembers Sue. "He worked with me, he knew how to ease the tension in my sore spots, and he gave me a lot of individual attention and therapy. About 60 percent of his work was helping me with passive exercises that were very painful at the time but in the long run eased the pain and tension in my upper body. Then for the other 40 percent he showed me how to do active exercises like working on the treadmill, strengthening my arm muscles, and doing some stretching exercises lying on a floor mat. I always felt better when I left."

Physical Therapy and Trigger Point Injections

Many people with FMS first see a physical therapist as adjunctive therapy along with trigger point injections. After your muscle knot is injected with medication to ease the pain, the physical therapist may gently massage the muscle and fascia to contribute to the release of trigger points and to enhance the effect of the medication. Although some spasmed muscles need trigger point injections, the goal should be eventually to manage the muscle problem with physical therapy alone and then at-home reconditioning exercises so your muscles no longer spasm and no longer need drug injections.

Toward the end of her therapy sessions, Sue found out how important the skill of the therapist can be. "There was another therapist," she says, "who took over in the last 2 weeks of my therapy, and I didn't like him at all. He showed me exercises and pointed me toward different types of equipment, but he didn't work with me personally, and I didn't feel any better each time I finished. I'm glad I didn't have him the entire time; I would have thought that therapy and exercise were useless."

After doing physical therapy and exercise three times a week for about six weeks, Sue left the supervised program and began her exercises alone at home. About 6 months later, she was given a gift certificate to a massage therapist. "I'm very sensitive to touch," says Sue. "If I'm even touched in certain areas, I feel pain, so I was unsure about trying massage." But she did, and the results have been good. "Once or twice a month, this woman does reflexology on my upper back and neck and helps the blood flow through the muscles," says Sue. "The massages are painful, but they seem to help a lot. This, along with sleeping well and exercising, seems to be all that I need right now."

For Sue, medication, physical therapy, at-home exercise, and therapeutic massages supply all the pain relief and energy she needs to enjoy her newborn daughter.

Avoid the Cookie Cutter

If you are lucky enough to find a good physical therapist who can teach you the exercises that will give you strength, endurance, flexibility, and pain relief, you will know what to do for yourself at home when the therapy sessions end. But what if you don't have this opportunity for professional guidance? Many people with fibromyalgia need to put together an exercise program on their own but wonder, "Where should I begin?"

This isn't an easy question to answer. Because there is no way of knowing your particular muscular state and your specific needs without a personal interview, you do not fit in a cookie-cutter program. The types of exercises best for you must be individualized, depending on personal choice and pain severity. This makes it very risky to offer a one-size-fits-all exercise program and expect it to help you reduce your symptoms of pain, fatigue, and sleep problems. A physical therapist should not do it, and a book on fibromyalgia should not do it. In this case, you're going to learn what's best for you by listening to your own body. Your body will tell you what is helping and what is not. Your body will tell you when you can do more and when you've done too much. It does take time, patience, and determination to build your own exercise program, but it can be done, and the benefits are worth the effort.

At-Home Exercises

Although your exercise program can't be prescribed step-by-step in this book, physical therapist Diane Scheufele, B.S., P.T., who is a team leader at the Fallon Clinic in Worcester, Massachusetts, for rehabilitation therapy, offers the following guiding principles on which to build your own program.

A Scientific Look at Fibromyalgia and Exercise

At the 64th Annual Scientific Meeting of the American College of Rheumatology held in Philadelphia in fall 2000, researchers from all over the world presented papers on the subject of fibromyalgia and exercise. A few of the studies and their conclusions are summarized here:

- **A randomized controlled study of strength training versus flexibility in fibromyalgia.** This study out of Portland, Oregon, consisted of a group of 68 women with FMS ages 28 to 59 who were assigned to a 12-week, twice-weekly exercise program consisting of either muscle strengthening or stretching. The study found that "it is feasible for fibromyalgia patients to take part in a specially tailored muscle-strengthening program and experience an improvement in overall disease activity, without a significant exercise induced flare in pain. Flexibility training alone also results in overall improvement, albeit of a lesser degree."[3]

- **Comparison of aerobic training and flexibility exercises for the treatment of fibromyalgia.** This study out of Brazil assigned 60 women with FMS between ages 18 and 65 to a 20-week exercise program of either aerobic exercises or flexibility exercises. In conclusion, "both exercise programs seem beneficial for patients with fibromyalgia; aerobic training was significantly better."[4]

- **A controlled trial of resistance training, cardiovascular and flexibility exercise on fitness, self-efficacy, and functional status in women with fibromyalgia.** In this study, 31 women from Boston with confirmed FMS exercised in groups three times a week for 1 hour per session. They were assessed before and after 20 weeks of exercise. The researchers concluded, "A program of progressive resistance training, cardiovascular and flexibility exercise can safely improve the fitness level, self-efficacy and functional status of women with FMS."[5]

- **Pool exercises combined with patient education for patients with fibromyalgia syndrome.** This study, composed of 59 people from Sweden with a mean age of 45 years and a mean symptom duration of 8.4 years, consisted of pool exercises for 6 months, combined with six sessions of patient education. The outcome showed significant improvements in the treatment group when it came to the assessment of the severity of the symptoms and consequences of FMS and the 6-minute walk test. These improvements could still be seen 6 months after the end of the program.[6]

- **A randomized controlled trial of exercise prescription for fibromyalgia.** This study of 136 patients in the United Kingdom evaluated the effect of a community-based exercise prescription program supervised by fitness instructors. In the end, both exercise and relaxation therapy were associated with significant improvements in tender point counts, all domains of FMS functioning, and improved employment status and reduced benefit claims. The benefits persisted at 1-year follow-up.[7]

- **Six-month and 1-year follow-up of fibromyalgia patients enrolled in a 23-week exercise program.** In this study, 416 FMS patients from Ontario, Canada, participated in a moderately intense exercise program of three, 30-minute classes per week for 23 weeks. In conclusion, the researchers found that "exercise, a simple and inexpensive intervention, can produce improvements in physical function, mood and self-efficacy for at least 12 months in patients who adhere to a 23 week program.[8]

Aerobic Exercises

"I generally don't tell people with fibromyalgia that they must do aerobic exercises," says Scheufele. "It's a nice goal, but 'exercising' doesn't necessarily have to mean working on a treadmill. The goal of exercise for this condition is to do what's necessary to continue working, doing daily chores, and having enough strength and flexibility to enjoy life. If aerobics is what you enjoy doing, great. Aerobics can be good because you can do a little bit of strengthening and get your blood flowing and get a release of certain chemicals that will ease pain. But you shouldn't put heavy expectations on yourself about how much aerobic exercise you 'should' be able to do.

"Many people with fibromyalgia are real pushers who want to do everything and do it all just right; they have a problem with learning to cope with the expectations they put on themselves. The fact that you can't run 3 miles a day anymore doesn't mean you can't gain benefit from a moderate exercise program. All you really should expect yourself to do is to move and keep moving."

Gentle-Motion Exercises

"A lot of the exercises I recommend for people with fibromyalgia who are just beginning an exercise program," says Scheufele, "are gentle, pain-free motion exercises to keep them moving, maybe just 2 minutes every hour. The exercise may be so slight that the person sitting next to you may not even notice that you're doing it." A few move-

---

Watch Out for the Cold

When exercising, be attentive to the air temperature. If you like to walk, try to do it in mild weather or on an indoor track; many people find that cold wind causes their FMS symptoms to flare. If you do water exercises, be aware that going from therapeutically warm water to the cooler air can cause muscles to tighten and ache.

ment exercises Scheufele recommends doing for 2 minutes at a time include the following:

- **For hips and lower back muscles.** From a sitting position with knees bent at a 90-degree angle and with both feet flat on the floor, slide one knee forward and the other knee back without moving in your seat. This will work your abdominal and hip muscles (but don't squeeze your buttocks). If you do this on and off throughout the day while you're working at a desk, let's say, you'll find that when you do stand up, your muscles won't hurt as much.

- **Spinal arch.** Put your weight on your elbows and lower arms as you place them on your desk or table from a sitting position. Round your spine up, and then arch it back, then forward and back. Don't move the elbows while you arch your back. In yoga this is called a *spinal flex*.

- **For relaxation.** Lie on the floor or on your bed. Bend your knees so your feet are flat on the ground. Rock both knees to the left and then to the right, but not so far that you'd call it a stretch. This is very relaxing to the nervous system.

Stretching Exercises

"People with fibromyalgia," says Scheufele, "need to make a habit of moving often and getting up and moving around." Try these simple stretching exercises to help keep yourself loose and flexible:

- **Spine and leg stretch.** Sit on the edge of your chair. Straighten one leg out in front of you, and straighten your spine so you're sitting up tall. This is a good stretch for your leg and spine. To increase the stretch, lean your body slightly forward from the hip. Hold the position for 20 to 30 seconds. Switch legs and repeat.

- **Neck stretch.** Slowly bring your ear toward your shoulder until you feel muscle tension in your neck. Breathe deeply and relax into the position. You should feel a gentle stretch, not a strain. Hold that position for about 30 seconds. Return your head to an upright position, repeat the exercise to the same side two or three times, and then repeat the exercise on the other side. This is a good stretch to do several times a day because a lot of people with fibromyalgia carry stress in their shoulders.

- **Hamstring stretch.** While standing, put your elbows on your desk or table, keeping your back and knees completely straight, so you have a 90-degree angle at your hips. Your toes must point straight ahead to get a good stretch. To get a better stretch, move your hips back further. You can do this while you talk on the phone or read your mail!

Postural Training

"During the day," says Scheufele, "if your head leans forward in front of your body, your line of gravity falls forward, and your whole back has to work to prevent you from falling on your face. That's one of the reasons that poor posture can aggravate the muscle tension that causes pain." These exercises will help you improve your daily posture.

- **Sit tall.** If you sit for long periods, you may find that you end up with a depressed sternum caused by a forward slouch in the upper back (some people call this the "computer position"). You need to sit tall, but don't just arch your back to do that—you'll put strain on the lower back. Instead, let the lower back slouch and lift up the breastbone as if you're suspended from the ceiling by a string attached to the top of your head.

- **Stand tall.** Stand with your back to a wall with your heels 2 to 4 inches away from the wall. Put as much of your body as possible flat against the wall to get your line of gravity behind your ankles where it belongs. This position reminds your body of how it should hold itself.

Strength Training

"There is value in strength training," says Scheufele, "because it increases muscle endurance and strength; and therefore, if you have a bad 2 or 3 days, it won't be so difficult to get back up and going again. But repetition is more important than weight, so you should begin with only 5 minutes of using lighter weights. Increase by adding another minute, not another 5 pounds. The hardest part is consistency; for strength training, you need to work at it two or three times a week."

Breathe Deeply

"Correct breathing while you exercise is very important," says Scheufele. "Blood and oxygen can't freely flow through your muscles if they're tense. So to oxygenate the tissues and get the maximum benefit from the time you put into exercising, you need to breathe correctly from the diaphragm." (See "Deep Breathing," page 132.)

How Much Exercise Is Enough?

All exercisers know that it's easy to push past the point of physical fatigue, but for the person with fibromyalgia, this practice can kill an exercise program. "When someone with fibromyalgia says to me, 'I can't exercise—it makes me feel worse,' I say it's not exercise that makes you feel worse; it's the way you're exercising," says Scheufele. "You have to know how to breathe correctly while you exercise and to pace yourself so you don't overdo it.

"Listen to your body," she adds. "If you are in pain after exercising, you'll know you did too much. But don't use that as an excuse to decide that exercise isn't good for you. Instead, be mindful of where your physical fatigue level is. Depending on how you feel, sometimes you will need to have an easier day. If you push on anyway, you may end up

At-Home Exercise Tips

When you build your own home-exercise program, remember these tips:

- Set goals that are small and attainable.

- Adjust your level of expectation to match what you are capable of doing in small steps.

- Move and gently stretch every few hours.

- Listen to your body and know when it is fatigued. If it hurts 2 hours after your workout, you did too much.

needing a late-day nap, which then throws off your sleep cycle, and then you make things worse all-around. That's why it's so important to set goals that are small and attainable. If you want to walk, fine. But don't start out expecting to go miles. Walk away from your house for 5 minutes, knowing it's going to take a little longer to return."

To find that type and amount of exercise that's just right for you, follow these guidelines:

- **Start slowly.** Sometimes you won't know for 24 hours whether what you're doing is too much. Start with one or two exercises on the first day for just a minute or two, and then see how you feel 24 hours later. If you're okay, then add another exercise or more time. Increase little by little staying in your comfort zone.

- **Pace yourself.** If you have been an active exerciser in the past, you will need to learn how to hold back, how to shake the old "no pain, no gain" philosophy. Rather than run until you drop, stop while you still feel okay and want to run again tomorrow.

- **Individualize.** Some people with fibromyalgia may enjoy walking 2 miles a day. Others may feel accomplished if they walk to the mailbox and back. Whatever intensity and frequency is best for you depends on how you feel and how you will feel tomorrow.

Be prepared to deal with slight postexercise pain. Take a pain reliever or use ice or heat after exercising to ease the soreness. But don't use a pain reliever before or during an exercise session—you won't be able to hear your body's signals that tell you when you've had enough.

Finding Relief in Warm-Water Exercises

Many people who have FMS say they feel like they've been run over by a car. Well, in Patty's case, she really was! After an accident 10 years ago, 57-year-old Patty began to feel achy and tired. These symptoms were blamed on menopause and the arthritis she had inherited from her parents. She was given prescription ibuprofen and sent on her way. However, after a few years of increasing discomfort and fatigue, Patty switched to a new doctor, who diagnosed her fibromyalgia, switched her to Celebrex (which was easier on her stomach), and prescribed physical therapy.

Although Patty wanted to exercise as her doctor had suggested, the physical therapy sessions hurt so badly and caused such great fatigue that she was useless for the rest of the day. "It may have been good for me," says Patty, "but it didn't make me feel good." As the pain increased, Patty was glad to be given Zoloft (an SSRI antidepressant) to treat the discomforts of menopause. Her doctor also prescribed trazodone (a tricyclic antidepressant) to help her sleep better. Unfortunately, the trazodone made Patty very drowsy in the morning and gave her a dry mouth, so she stopped taking it and was left with pain and fatigue.

Then something happened that was a turning point for Patty. "I read about a water exercise class for people with arthritis and thought I'd give that a try," remembers Patty. "And I'm so glad I did. Doing exercises in water that is 91 degrees makes me feel the best out of everything I've tried." Patty also swims in her neighborhood pool, which is not heated, but she doesn't enjoy it as much. "Any kind of swimming is good therapy, I'm sure," she says, "but after swimming in a cold-water pool, I don't feel as good afterward as I do when I exercise in the warmer water."

Having arthritis, Patty noticed an announcement for this swim program created specifically for people with arthritis, but she is sure it is doing a world of good for the aches and pains of fibromyalgia, too. "Most of the people in my class are 80-year-olds, but I don't care," she laughs. "Getting in the water and moving without feeling any stiffness or pain is just wonderful and invigorating. I feel good for the rest of the day. Then I feel like getting out and doing something. I'm able to exercise my muscles without having pain and fatigue during and afterward. The instructor helps us slowly move every part of the body from fingers to toes without exertion for about 30 minutes. I don't know what this will do for me long-term, but I know it makes the world of difference for me now. My lower back pain has really improved; I can just feel those muscles strengthening."

Patty's right. Many people with fibromyalgia find warm-water aerobics help them enjoy exercise and reap the benefits. You can probably find a warm-water program by calling local hospitals, universities, and pain clinics that have rehabilitation programs. Ask if they have warm-water exercise programs. The classes may be advertised for people with arthritis, but they are also very helpful for learning to exercise with the pain of fibromyalgia.

SIT DOWN AND RELAX

Research strongly supports what you probably already know: Stress aggravates the symptoms of fibromyalgia. What happens physically in your body during periods of stress is really quite dramatic and has the power to make you feel absolutely miserable. Here's why.

The roots of the body's physical response to stress go back to our primitive days. In the era of cave people, the difference between bringing an animal home to eat and being eaten by the animal was a person's ability to react quickly to danger. The human body had to be able to prepare for fight or flight at a moment's notice. To do this, the sympathetic portion of the autonomic nervous system of the body sent norepinephrine neurons out that influence all major organs and cause the release of adrenaline (epinephrine) from the adrenal glands. Adrenaline causes rapid heart rate, dry mouth, increased blood pressure, dilated pupils, sweating, redirection of blood flow to the muscles and away from the digestive tract and skin (causing the pale look of terror), and muscle tremor.

> *What happens physically in your body during periods of stress is really quite dramatic and has the power to make you feel absolutely miserable.*

The problem is that this stress response, which was designed to promote the physical activity of running away or fighting, is no longer appropriate for us today. When we are stuck in traffic and late for an appointment, we do not need extra oxygen directed to our deep muscles, and yet it happens. Even with no foe in sight and nowhere to run, our heart beats rapidly, our blood pressure rises, and our muscles tighten.

To add to this body assault, during the stress response a complex process causes the release of the stress hormone cortisol into the bloodstream. Cortisol can cause a simple stressful situation to have negative consequences on the body, lasting from several hours to weeks and months if the stress is repeated and chronic (e.g., having widespread muscular pain).

Initially, cortisol release during stress has several good purposes. It suppresses the immune system, which if you are in a fight (or running from a predator) keeps a small injury from swelling up, preventing you from fighting back or getting away. Cortisol also causes the level of blood sugar to rise, making it more available for use in the brain and muscles for energy and quick action. Cortisol reaches the brain and, acutely, acts as a stimulant, heightening your sense of awareness.

In the long run, however, the release of cortisol in severe or chronic stress will take an undesirable toll on the body. In animals, the long-term exposure to stress beyond the animal's control, or in a repeated fashion, results in a depression-like syndrome called "learned helplessness," in which the animal loses drive, interacts less with other animals, becomes slower in movement, and eventually even dies. In the brains of such animals, release of cortisol becomes continuous. Neurons that release cortisol remain activated for extended periods, causing burnout or depression.[9]

> *Letting stress go unchecked is like supercharging your FMS.*

The constant release of adrenaline and cortisol that's caused by unrelenting stress of both daily life and chronic pain fuels the symptoms of fibromyalgia. Letting stress go unchecked is like supercharging your FMS. That's why relaxation exercises are an important part of any treatment program for this syndrome.

The Power of Relaxation

Reducing stress reduces pain in several ways:

- Relaxation exercises can control the involuntary workings of the nervous system that are known to support and aggravate pain. These techniques can help you manage pain by influencing blood pressure, heart rate, respiration, and metabolism— all seemingly involuntary physiological functions that power the chronic pain cycle.

- Relaxation exercises enhance the quality of sleep. Relaxation techniques calm the body, improve circulation, and lower anxiety levels—all of which promote peaceful rest.

- Relaxation therapy reduces the sensation of pain by decreasing muscle tension.

- Relaxation techniques reduce anxiety. It's difficult to think positively and continue your pain-management regimen each day if you are chronically anxious and tense.

- Relaxation exercises improve your sense of control over pain. They put you in charge; they give you an active role in managing your pain. This reduces the feelings of helplessness and hopelessness that support and maintain pain.

Eric Willmarth, Ph.D., who is president of the Michigan Behavioral Consultants (MBC) and director of behavioral medicine for the Pain Management Center at Holland Community Hospital in Michigan, has a special interest in helping people with FMS learn how to relax. He says, "The most direct way in which stress affects the pain of fibromyalgia is through the instinctive reaction to guard and brace. We tense our muscles up and hold our bodies in certain postures, which does sometimes give some relief in a specific area but causes bigger problems in the long run. Chronic pain conditions tend to lead to chronic muscle tension. This causes the muscles to use more energy and fatigue—both adding to the level of pain—creating a vicious cycle. Also, the longer you tense up, the more likely you are to cause the muscles to physically shorten and cut down on your range of motion and flexibility."

In addition to the muscle tension caused by the guard-and-brace reaction to pain, people with fibromyalgia are also subject to the same daily tensions as everyone else that add to muscle tension. Dr. Willmarth agrees that if you have a 45-minute commute to work in congested traffic and find yourself gripping the steering wheel with white knuckles, you are further aggravating an already-difficult medical condition. "And," he adds, "no matter how hard you squeeze the wheel it's not going to add any energy to the car or make you go any faster, so it's wasted energy that people with fibromyalgia can't afford to give away. But a person who knows how to use some simple relaxation techniques could use that 45 minutes as an opportunity to increase body energy and ease pain."

To use relaxation techniques most effectively, you have to begin to listen to your body and understand how, where, and when you hold onto tension. You have to know that a trip to the dentist can throw you into an FMS flare if you're the kind of patient who grips your seat and tenses your entire body while in the dentist's chair. You have to learn to recognize what muscle tension feels like and then learn how to relax. "We each have a certain pool of energy each day," says Dr. Willmarth. "The stress habits we unconsciously practice are a leak in that pool, and people with fibromyalgia are quick to pay the consequences. We need to become more efficient with the energy we've got and not allow stress to rob us of any."

> *To use relaxation techniques most effectively, you have to begin to listen to your body and understand how, where, and when you hold onto tension.*

"But," cautions Dr. Willmarth, "telling someone to 'just relax' is like telling her to 'just speak German.' For someone who did not grow up speaking German and never learned it in school, such advice is ridiculous. The advice 'just relax' is equally ridiculous to people who do not know how. Relaxation is a skill just like any other skill that needs time and practice to perfect."

When you use the relaxation techniques explained later in this section, Dr. Willmarth advises that you do them in ways that are easy and, of course, "relaxing." "The worst thing people can do," says Dr. Willmarth, "is to start off thinking, 'I have to put aside 45 minutes tonight to relax,' or 'I have to make time to follow this hour-long relaxation tape and do all the things it tells me.' Even if they make it through a few sessions, they spend most of the time jumping out of their skin and quickly decide that relaxation isn't for them. I would much rather have someone begin by practicing a relaxation technique for 1 or 2 minutes in the beginning just to get an idea of the value of a relaxed feeling."

Here are a few relaxation techniques recommended by Dr. Willmarth that you can use to get you started as you learn to change the way your body handles the stress of pain and everyday life.

Deep Breathing

People with fibromyalgia (as well as many other people in stressful situations) tend to breathe with their chest muscles. If you take a deep breath right now, you may find that your chest puffs out as you fill your lungs with air—this breathing habit is adding to your pain and fatigue! Watch a child as he sleeps and you'll see the stomach muscles rise with each breath as the diaphragm—not the chest—fills with air. Many adults have lost this natural breathing mechanism that is most efficient in bringing restorative oxygen to all tissues of the body.

Every day, practice breathing from your diaphragm:

1. Place one hand on your chest and one on your stomach.

2. As you take a deep breath in, feel the hand on your stomach rise. The hand on your chest should not rise up.

3. Let the air go. Don't push it out. Let it go gently. Feel the hand on your stomach go down.

When you have the knack of diaphragm breathing, focus on the pace of your breathing. Short, shallow breaths are stressful to the body. As you practice this deep breathing technique, change your pace to six breaths per minute. (If you check your "natural" breathing pattern right now, you may find that you're taking about 10 breaths per minute.) Take in a slow easy breath to the count of four. Then release the breath to the count of four. Hold your breath for 2 seconds. This 10-second cycle will give you six breaths per minute.

Deep breathing is a strategy you can use anywhere. No one around needs to know you're practicing a stress-reduction technique. It's a technique you can engage in whenever you feel your pain increasing and your body tensing. Automatically, deep breathing will change your body's reaction to pain.

In the beginning, you'll find that although the deep breathing exercise is easy, your chest-breathing habit will return as soon as you're not paying attention. Give yourself a couple of weeks of practicing deep breathing just a few minutes here and there throughout the day, and soon you'll find that your body will relearn how to breathe correctly on its own.

Mental Imagery

To feel pain, your brain has to perceive it. Mental imagery literally takes your mind off your pain and focuses it on something positive, causing the brain to release brain chemicals that elevate mood and diminish pain—really!

Dr. Willmarth suggests you give this quick example of the power of mental imagery a try: Close your eyes and imagine a large, yellow lemon. Now picture the lemon being cut into quarters, and imagine biting into one of the quarters. What happens? Even though there was no actual lemon, many people will find the simple exercise enough to cause their lips to pucker and their mouths to water. This is a good example of how the mind's ability to picture something can set off certain physiological reactions.

> *The goal with mental imagery for relaxation is to ease the muscle tension of stress by tricking the body into thinking you're relaxed and having a good time.*

The goal with mental imagery for relaxation is to ease the muscle tension of stress by tricking the body into thinking you're relaxed and having a good time. Sit back, close your eyes, and imagine a very pleasant incident or place. For example, some people find this kind of image soothing:

> I am stretched out on the ocean beach. The sun is warm on my body. When it gets too strong, I have an umbrella for protection. I feel the warmth of the sand on my fingertips. I see the calm ocean touching the shore. I can smell the salt of the ocean, and I can taste the sea air. On my beach there's just the right number of people—I'm not crowded or lonely. On my beach there are no sand crabs or flies. I feel just wonderful. It's an ideal place that I can visit with all my senses anytime I want. Even when I'm in the middle of a crowd with my eyes wide open, I can go to my beach.

This safe place happens to be a beach—yours can be anywhere. It can be in your family room by the fireplace, the woods by a stream, the park down the street. It can be anywhere, but keep these pointers in mind:

- **Make the place real.** When you're stressed or in pain, you won't be able to relate to an alien planet.

- **Involve all of your senses.** Make sure all the smells and the things you touch, taste, hear, and see in this environment are pleasing to you.

- **Go to this place often.** The more you practice increasing the quality of your image, the more you can rely on it when you're in pain. It will become a practiced response.

Progressive Muscle Relaxation

In stressful situations, many people describe the way they feel as being "tied up in knots." Because of the way our muscles react to stress, this actually is true. Progressive muscle relaxation will help you untie the knots by teaching you how to recognize muscle tension and then how to relax the involved muscles. Then, when you feel stress in physical pain, you can relax those muscles that are aggravating your pain. By practicing progressive muscle relaxation, you will learn what it feels like when stress begins to manifest itself in muscle tension. Then when your muscles do begin to tense involuntarily, you will be able to identify the problem area and stop the stress attack.

To begin, tense and relax a muscle group—let's start with your right hand and arm. Press your forearm down against the table. Feel where the tension goes out through your fingertips, up into your shoulder, right into your neck. Maintain that tension for 5 to 10 seconds so you

> *Progressive muscle relaxation will help you untie the knots by teaching you how to recognize muscle tension and then how to relax the involved muscles.*

have time to feel how whole parts of your body are involved in tension. Then relax. Feel the experience of letting go—of consciously relaxing your muscles. Then move on to other muscle groups; do this exercise with each leg and foot, the abdomen and chest, the face, jaw, and forehead. By repeating this exercise muscle group by muscle group throughout the body, you develop more and more control over the muscles and become increasingly sensitive and attuned to how a tense muscle and a relaxed muscle feels. Frequent repetition of short practice times throughout the day is a good way to learn this skill.

When you're comfortable with these basics, go on to explore other types of relaxation strategies. There is no strategy created specifically for fibromyalgia; anything you find that leads you to a relaxed state will improve your overall pain state. You can find various types of relaxation programs on the bookshelves. (The classic in this field is Dr. Herbert Benson's *The Relaxation Response* [Berkley Publishing Group, 1994].) You can buy relaxation audio- and videotapes that walk you through the steps of various exercises. Or you can sign up to take a class in more advanced types of relaxation techniques that may require some guidance and supervision to use them effectively like yoga and meditation.

Qi Gong Meditation

Many different types of meditation can effectively help you relax and reduce muscle tension. The ancient Chinese healing art of Qi Gong (also written as Chi Kung and Chi Gong) is a form that is gaining popularity among people with fibromyalgia because of its ability to calm the body as well as ease pain.

Qi Gong teacher Paddy Kennedy (who herself has fibromyalgia and teaches Qi Gong classes to people with FMS) explains: "Qi Gong is the art and skill of moving one's vital energy throughout the entire body—almost like administering your own acupuncture treatment. Once we have learned how to move this energy throughout our body, we are able to attain the three principal goals of Qi Gong practice: relaxation, tranquility, and the ability to go with the flow of nature (learning to relax and accept the things in the world that we cannot change). As soon as we enter into a state of tranquility, our bodies automatically begin to make tranquilizer-type chemicals that help to soothe pain and repair damaged cells and tissue.

"Perhaps the most helpful aspect of Qi Gong practice for the person with FMS, though, is its analgesic capability," Kennedy adds. "Practicing Qi Gong produces, in the brain and intestinal walls, large amounts of enkephalin and stimulates the body's morphine receptors to accept the enkephalin easily. The pain-relieving effect of enkephalin is many times more effective than that of morphine.

Qi Gong is gaining popularity among people with fibromyalgia because of its ability to calm the body as well as ease pain.

"There are two distinct forms of Qi Gong: the active or standing form and the passive or sitting form," she explains. "It is my strong belief that the passive form of Qi Gong is better for people with FMS because it does not require standing in uncomfortable poses for long periods of time, nor does it require a great deal of memory of what comes next. Sitting or passive Qi Gong is a guided meditation that can be done lying down, sitting on a chair or on a cushion on the floor. It is gentle, soothing, relaxing, and healing."

Author Miryam Ehrlich Williamson finds that sitting Qi Gong is one of the mainstays of her program for dealing with her fibromyalgia. "I met Paddy Kennedy at a fibromyalgia conference in New York City in 1997," says Miryam (who is the author of *The Fibromyalgia Relief Book* [Walker, 1998]). "Since that time, I've been doing Qi Gong by following her CD. I admit that I don't do my meditation as often as I would like to, but the two or three times a week that I do it are wonderful for my body. All I need is a comfortable straight-back chair and no interruptions. Then I use a CD player with headphones and let Patty's soothing voice guide me through the exercise. That's all there is to it.

"Qi Gong has taught me to visualize energy coming into my body, moving through the body, and leaving," says Miryam. "I'm not very adept at visualization, but I have come to the point where I can see my qi (my energy)."

The focus on breathing during this meditation has been especially helpful to Miryam. "People with fibromyalgia are often shallow breathers, and I believe that a considerable portion of my discomfort comes from faulty breathing," she says. Miryam knows the value of proper breathing because she is a singer. "I'd noticed for years that I always felt better after I had been rehearsing. Now I believe it was the correct breathing patterns I used while singing that filled my body with the oxygen it needed. Qi Gong has taught me to breathe much better—although I still find when I'm busy at work, I forget to breathe deeply. So I have a sign over my desk that says, 'Breathe!'"

Like many others, Miryam finds meditation especially helpful when she is stressed. "When I know I'm stressed and my body is pumping adrenaline, I know I'm going to be sick afterward," she says. "So as soon as I can, I get to Qi Gong. Even if I don't have the CD with me, I'll sit down and do the breathing and visualization that I can remember. The physical act of doing that seems to burn off some of that adrenaline that I know otherwise is going to back up and make me feel ill. It is a tremendous way of saving myself from post-stress malaise. So for me, this meditation is both curative and preventative."

But Miryam is quick to point out that for her, meditation is not religious. "I think there are people who are skittish about meditation because they think of it as a religious observance that may conflict with their own religion," she says. "That hesitation comes from a misunderstanding of what meditation is. For me it is not a religious function at all. It's a physical activity; just like my morning workouts are necessary to my well-being, so is meditation. It has nothing to do with religion."

When finished with her meditation, Miryam says she experiences a feeling of peace and of softened muscles. "Although I have no scientific basis for this," she says, "the results of meditation make me think that some of the tension in my muscles comes from lack of oxygen. When I meditate, I'm practically floating afterward; I have no muscle tension. I honestly believe that for most people with fibromyalgia, simply learning to sit still, and be, and breathe deeply offers tremendous benefits."

You can order Paddy Kennedy's CD entitled *Qi Gong for Chronic Pain Management* by e-mail at paddyk@bestweb.net.

Biofeedback

"One of the biggest problems with using relaxation exercises effectively," says Dr. Willmarth, "is that we are not very tuned into our bodies, and we don't know when we're tense and when we're not tense." That's why many people with fibromyalgia find biofeedback very helpful.

Biofeedback measures muscle tension by measuring the amount of electrical activity going through the muscles. Dr. Willmarth explains:

> Biofeedback doesn't do anything to you. It just gives you information. It helps you "see" your muscle tension and "see" how relaxation exercises can reduce the tension that contributes to your pain.
>
> We know that 1 to 3 microvolts is a good resting level for muscle tension. I can't tell you how often I've had people sitting in the chair at 20 or 30 microvolts assuring me that they are very relaxed. They don't remember anymore what it feels like to be relaxed. With biofeedback, I can hook them up to the computer and show them the levels of tension and how they can control those levels with relaxation exercises. With progressive muscle relaxation exercises, for example, they can tense a muscle group, see the tension level rise on the computer, and then relax the muscle and see the level fall. They can visually see the difference. We also see the tension level rise if I tell a person to "try to relax." That becomes work and tension rises, but if you learn to "let" yourself relax, you'll see the positive result—you'll learn to automatically adjust the way you let your body hold on to tension. Often a person who learns to relax muscles and keep them relaxed at a lower level of tension

> **Referral Resource**
>
> To find a biofeedback practitioner near you, contact:
>
> **Association of Applied Psychophysiology and Biofeedback (AAPB)**
> Phone: (303) 422-8436
> Web site: www.aapb.org

finds out that it's hard work to tighten their muscles to reach the level of tension their bodies used to hold on to naturally.

Stress Alert

While you're learning to release the muscle tension caused by stress, you should also help your body avoid this tension to begin with by learning to reduce the amount of stress you expose yourself to each day. No one can eliminate stress completely (and who would want to live such a boring life!), but you can be on the alert for situations and people who tend to fill you with stress. If you know that a trip to the amusement park with your kids and their four friends will push you over the edge—don't go! If you know that a coworker's constant complaining and negative attitude make you feel tense—avoid her! If your job is so hectic and pressured that you feel you're about to explode every day of your life—think seriously about finding another job. As someone with fibromyalgia, the quality of your daily life can be severely affected by the amount of stress you have to deal with. So take an inventory of where excessive stress may be coming from, and do something to change the situation. This is one area of your treatment plan that you have the power to control. Take a deep breath right now and promise yourself that you are going to do yourself the favor of avoiding stressful people and places.

Take an inventory of where excessive stress may be coming from, and do something to change the situation. This is one area of your treatment plan that you have the power to control.

Medication, exercise, and relaxation strategies are the foundation of most treatment programs for fibromyalgia. Scientific research studies and the personal experiences of many people with fibromyalgia testify to their value in treating the pain and fatigue of this illness. However, many find that other complementary and alternative treatment therapies also help them live with this chronic condition. Chapter 5 will give you a peek at some of these most popular therapies.

CHAPTER 5

The Mind-Body Connection

Y OU'RE TAKING YOUR medication. You're exercising as best you can. You've started working on some relaxation techniques. But still you have a nagging, ominous feeling that just maybe the doctors, your colleagues, and some of your friends and family may be right—maybe this really is the "AIYH" syndrome (short for "all in your head!") So many "experts" may have already told you that there is nothing physically wrong with you. People have quizzically remarked, "But you look so healthy." And you do have some good days that make you wonder about the reality of the really bad days. Maybe you are beginning to think that the mind-body connection you keep hearing about is to blame for all your symptoms. Whoa! Before you let yourself go down that road, keep reading.

In this chapter you'll be assured that although there is a strong mind-body connection in the experience of fibromyalgia, that does not mean that FMS is "all in your head." It means that your symptoms of pain and fatigue (which have a very real basis in physiological dysfunction) can be worsened or improved by the way you think about your condition. It means that stress, negative emotions, and attitudes can influence how you experience FMS, but they do not cause it. It means that any chronic condition can lead to depression but that the condition is not the result of the depression. You need to know more about these facts to make sure that the mind-body relationship in this illness works for you, not against you.

FIGHTING THE AIYH SYNDROME

Despite increasing research distinguishing FMS from psychiatric disorders, the role of psychological factors in this illness is still being hotly debated. As you probably are well aware, many medical professionals still firmly believe that fibromyalgia is nothing more than a problem of stress, anxiety, or depression. But, fortunately, many others staunchly advocate the physical disease basis of this illness. Nationally renowned FMS expert Muhammad B. Yunus, M.D., argues that while psychological factors may aggravate symptoms, they are not the cause (which he believes, as described in chapter 1, involves a dysfunction in the central nervous system). Dr. Yunus believes that the physicians who cling to the belief that FMS is a psychological disorder suffer themselves from "disturbed physician syndrome" (DPS). With great passion, Dr. Yunus says, "DPS people are trouble because of their preoccupation that FMS patients are psychologically disturbed. It is not the FMS patients who are disturbed; it is the physicians who are psychologically disturbed because they ignore the data, and whatever data there is, they manipulate it to say what they want it to say."[1]

Fortunately, support for a fair and understanding assessment of your illness is growing nationwide. A presenter at the Fibromyalgia Awareness Main Event (FAME) 2000 International Fibromyalgia Conference boldly asserted, "Given the amount of research that shows physical abnormalities in fibromyalgia, anyone who still believes this

> *Stress, negative emotions, and attitudes can influence how you experience FMS, but they do not cause it.*

> **Not All in Your Head!**
>
> The next time someone suggests that FMS is all in your head, remind that person that people with arthritis and multiple sclerosis were also once told their symptoms were manifestations of psychological stress. The fact that the exact cause of FMS has not yet been discovered does not mean that it doesn't exist.

illness is 'all in your head' should have *their* head examined!"[2] This is good reason to hope that in the very near future no one will have to struggle to convince the world that FMS is a very real illness.

The Frustration of the Somatization Label

The November 13, 2000, edition of *The New Yorker* ran an article called "Hurting All Over: With So Many People in So Much Pain, How Could Fibromyalgia Not Be a Disease?" Although the title offered hope that fibromyalgia would receive deserved attention, sadly the article spent undue time reinforcing the AIYH syndrome theory. The author talked with two doctors who are self-described "opponents of the current treatment of fibromyalgia": Dr. Thomas Bohr, a neurologist at the Loma Linda University School of Medicine, and Dr. Arthur Barsky, a psychiatry professor at Harvard University.

According to the article, the two doctors "contend that even honoring this bundle of symptoms with a medical label may be doing more to make people sick than to cure them." The rationale used for this claim is that everyone—even healthy people—has aches and pains and fatigue. Dr. Barsky believes that for patients diagnosed with fibromyalgia, these everyday symptoms become a focus of increased attention. Says Barsky, "they become trapped in the belief that their symptoms are due to disease, with future expectations of debility and doom." This is a mind-body relationship associated with fibromyalgia that makes it almost impossible to get appropriate treatment from physicians who do not believe your disease is real.

It is not hard to understand why some physicians label fibromyalgia as a psychological ailment. After all, medical doctors are trained to diagnose illness based on concrete test results. If a doctor is not familiar with or trained to administer the tender point exam for fibromyalgia (which the majority of doctors are not), he or she can not see a neat diagnostic pattern. In that case, the doctor may go to a diagnostic label learned in medical school called *somatization*, or better known to people with fibromyalgia as the "there's nothing really wrong with you" diagnosis. This doesn't mean this is a "bad" doctor, just an uninformed (or stubborn) one.

The doctor may go to a diagnostic label called somatization, *or better known as the "there's nothing really wrong with you" diagnosis. This doesn't mean this is a "bad" doctor, just an uninformed (or stubborn) one.*

A recent article in the leading journal for primary care doctors called the *American Family Physician* says, "Patients who somatize present with persistent physical complaints for which a physiologic explanation cannot be found."[3] How easy it would be to lump fibromyalgia into that category? Further along in the article, physicians are reminded of the diagnostic features that suggest somatization. They are multiple symptoms (often occurring in different organ systems), symptoms that are vague or exceed objective findings, chronic course, presence of a psychiatric disorder, history of extensive diagnostic testing, and rejection of previous physicians. If you have fibromyalgia, most or even all of these criteria may describe you! That's why a doctor who has never studied fibromyalgia in medical school and who can find no conclusive evidence of disease through standard testing will scribble "somatization" on your chart and send you off with some kind of antidepressant or tranquilizer to help you calm down and better deal with stress.

Certainly, there is such a thing as somatization. Some people do experience physical symptoms in response to stress, and some do complain of pain and illness because they crave attention. Some of these people may even have FMS, but that doesn't mean FMS is automatically a form of somatization! If you read further in this article, you'll find that "the somatizing patient seems to seek the sick role, which affords relief from stressful or impossible interpersonal expectations ('primary gain') and, in most societies, provides attention, caring, and sometimes even monetary reward ('secondary gain'). This is not malingering (consciously 'faking' the symptoms), because the patient is not aware of the process through which the symptoms arise, cannot will them away, and genuinely suffers from the symptoms."[4]

The medical mind-set that the symptoms of fibromyalgia match the criteria for somatization encourages many physicians to ignore the volumes of scientific facts and make a quick and easy diagnosis of psychological disorder. That's why choosing the right physician is *so* important.

A Long Journey Through the AIYH Syndrome

Thirty-seven-year-old Donna is a quality assessment improvement systems coordinator for a mental health and mental retardation organization; she also has fibromyalgia and a wonderful doctor who understands exactly what she is going through. But it was not always this way. Donna spent 3 years with a family doctor who persistently assured her that her pain and fatigue were caused by stress. "There were days when the bottoms of my feet would hurt so much that I couldn't walk," remembers Donna. "And there were days when I couldn't even comb my hair because it hurt so much. I had extreme headaches and body aches all over. I was in unbelievable pain. My doctor said I was overdoing it and I should slow down. With two young children, that wasn't going to happen, but he was sure that the stress of being a mother was causing the pain and fatigue that I was complaining about."

Like many physicians, when the symptoms persisted and grew worse, Donna's doctor tried to pin the cause on depression. "He gave me the antidepressant Zoloft, but I really didn't want it. I'm an extremely optimistic person and knew I wasn't at all depressed. But he felt that I just didn't know I was depressed. I would argue and argue, but he insisted that I give it a try. All the medication did was make me feel like a dysfunctional zombie. But still the doctor felt I should give it more time to work. He also wanted me to do stress-reduction exercises like visual imagery. I also went through dream analysis in case bad dreams were keeping me from getting a good night's sleep. (Staying awake is my real problem, not falling asleep, but he said I probably didn't realize that I wasn't sleeping soundly.) Part of me wanted to believe that all of my symptoms were stress related, but I just knew that stress alone couldn't make me hurt as much as I was hurting."

Then Donna moved and found a new doctor—but her troubles weren't over just yet. "This was a female rheumatologist who I hoped would be a little more compassionate. But when I complained that the antidepressants she put me on made me cry all day, she became very frustrated and said, 'I don't know what's wrong with you, but I do think that you should see a psychiatrist.'" Donna didn't go to a psychiatrist but did find a new doctor. "He is a wonderful man who knew exactly what I had and how to best help me work with it. I've been with him for 2 years, and I'm doing so much better now." Unfortunately, Donna has recently changed health insurance companies and can no longer go to this doctor, so her search for a knowledgeable physician now begins again.

THE TRUTH ABOUT DEPRESSION AND FIBROMYALGIA

As if being accused of faking illness and milking sympathy with pain weren't bad enough, some people with fibromyalgia also have to deal with the long-held belief, "There's nothing physically wrong with you; you're just depressed." Or equally as maddening, "You have fibromyalgia because you're depressed." This assumption that depression and fibromyalgia are one and the same thing is totally false but still hangs tough in many medical circles. FMS and depression can be related, but not in the way that allows some doctors to use depression as their scapegoat.

You, yourself, may see a connection: You know you have very real chronic widespread pain, sleep disturbances, and debilitating fatigue (for starters). You know there is no cure right now, and you don't know how you'll be able to function tomorrow—it's no wonder you may feel down, anxious, and upset! In fact, it would be abnormal if you did not feel mentally and emotionally awful. And there's no doubt that persistent pain and unrelieved misery can sometimes lead to clinical depression, but that does not mean your fibromyalgia symptoms should ever be dismissed as "just depression." The disease of depression is entirely separate from the disease of fibromyalgia. So why do some healthcare professionals insist, "You're not really sick; you're just depressed," as if you couldn't possibly be both sick *and* depressed or have an illness that has symptoms similar to depression but that is not depression at all? As with most issues concerning fibromyalgia, the answer is not simple.

> *This assumption that depression and fibromyalgia are one and the same thing is totally false but still hangs tough in many medical circles.*

As discussed briefly in chapter 1, because nearly one-third of people with fibromyalgia has a history of depression before being diagnosed with FMS, medical professionals used to believe that depression was the cause of this condition. But today, the American College of Rheumatology has created standard diagnostic criteria that confirm FMS as a true illness and not merely psychological in nature. And new studies have shown that people with fibromyalgia are no more depressed than those with other chronic, painful, and debilitating disorders, such as rheumatoid arthritis. There's no doubt that people with fibromyalgia live in circumstances that can trigger depression, but in his 1994 study of fibromyalgia syndrome, Dr. Yunus states definitively, "It is clear that abnormal psychological status is not a requirement for development of fibromyalgia."[5]

Other scientific research supports Dr. Yunus's claim. It has been proven beyond a doubt that depression and fibromyalgia are two separate conditions—some medical professionals just don't get it yet, but they will. It's hard to ignore facts like these:

> *F*ibromyalgia symptoms should never be dismissed as "just depression." The disease of depression is entirely separate from the disease of fibromyalgia.

- The vast majority of patients with fibromyalgia do not meet criteria for a current psychiatric diagnosis.[6]

- People with FMS and depression who are treated for depression generally respond well to antidepressant medications, yet the symptoms of pain and disordered sleep continue.[7]

- Not all people with FMS also have depression. Those who do sometimes suffered depression before the onset of fibromyalgia; others become depressed after the onset of fibromyalgia.[8]

- People with fibromyalgia are no more depressed than other patients with chronic rheumatic diseases such as rheumatoid arthritis.[9]

Findings like these are beginning to erase the "psychological" label that has kept many people with fibromyalgia from receiving appropriate treatment, but not everyone has gotten the word. Many people with fibromyalgia still fight this battle with uninformed physicians. Twenty-four-year-old Ahmie is a special education teacher who has a bachelor's degree in psychology and sociology and is working toward a master's degree in education. She has done all of this despite the fact that she has had the symptoms of FMS since she was 10 years old. At that time she was told her aches and pains were only "growing pains," and when she continued to complain, she was called a hypochondriac. Finally, at age 17 she received the correct diagnosis of FMS, but her trouble getting doctors to listen to her was just beginning.

"My current doctor first met with me for 5 minutes and decided I was depressed," Ahmie says. "I told her, 'Honey, I've had FMS for more than half my life; I'm over the depression part.' Then she announced that I was bipolar, but I knew that couldn't be right. (I have a degree in psychology and know the diagnostic criteria for bipolar disorder.) I tried to tell this doctor that I'm depressed maybe part of one day per month, usually around my period, but that information didn't interest her. She then tried to tell me that I was manic. By then I had had it with her obsession with tagging a psychological illness on me. I told her to try telling me that again after she got a Ph.D. in psychology or psychiatry."

The vast majority of patients with fibromyalgia do not meet criteria for a current psychiatric diagnosis.

The doctor's response was to hand Ahmie a prescription for the SSRI antidepressant Paxil. "She gave me this prescription even though I told her that the last time I was on an SSRI (Zoloft, in particular), it caused insomnia, migraines, and periods of unresponsiveness, which were probably petite mal seizures (although I never pursued a diagnosis because I could tell when they were coming and didn't want to lose my then-newly-acquired driver's license). I've seen this doctor two times since that first infuriating visit. Both times she has asked how the Paxil was working, and both times I've told her, 'Couldn't tell ya, 'cause I'm not taking it.' She just shrugs and goes on with the exam. I have a feeling that she thinks *I'm* being difficult." Like many doctors who are ill equipped to treat fibromyalgia, it sounds like Ahmie's doctor hasn't kept up on the latest facts.

This insistence on tying fibromyalgia to depression might have been unavoidable years ago, but it shouldn't happen today. "It was easy for doctors to attribute the pain to psychological disorders," says Lawrence Bradley, Ph.D., professor of medicine in the Division of Clinical Immunology and Rheumatology at the University of Alabama at Birmingham, who is also a psychiatrist. "That perception is beginning to change now that we can show distinctly different brain function that is not evident in patients with depression."[10]

Dr. Bradley's insights are backed by studies that have found that certain markers of depression are not present in all people with fibromyalgia. In particular, when studying why some patients with fibromyalgia are depressed and some others are not, assistant professor Akiko Okifuji, Ph.D., and his colleagues from the University of Washington in Seattle concluded that there is not enough evidence to say that fibromyalgia and depression share a common mechanism. Laboratory findings using the dexamethasone suppression test, a marker for major depression, have been reported as normal in patients with FMS. And normal or decreased 24-hour urinary cortisol levels have been reported in patients with FMS, whereas depressed patients had significantly higher cortisol levels than both patients with FMS and healthy persons.[11]

Treating Depression As a Separate Illness

Despite these definitive differences, there's no doubt that some people with fibromyalgia are also clinically depressed. The danger in this situation comes from the assumption that the two naturally go together and can be treated the same. In the article, "Depression in People with Chronic Illness," depression specialist Arthur Rifkin, M.D., a psychiatrist at Albert Einstein Medical Center in New York, offers this word of warning: "The most common misconception about depression and chronic illness is that it's understandable to become depressed when faced with a chronic illness. It is understandable—but only during the initial adjustment period that should not last for more than a few months. Beyond that, persistent depression should be treated as a separate illness."[12]

If you know you have fibromyalgia and depression or if you have fibromyalgia and wonder whether you might also have depression, fibromyalgia medical advocates strongly urge you to see the two as separate medical entities and seek appropriate treatment for *both*—especially in view of the way they each can influence the other:

- The depression caused by chronic illnesses often aggravates the illness. This is especially true in the case of fibromyalgia because it is well known that depression makes pain hurt more. It causes fatigue and lethargy that can exacerbate the loss of energy caused by the FMS, and it can further interfere with social functioning because depression tends to make people withdraw into social isolation.

- Depression impairs the immune system, which can hurt the body's efforts to combat illness. In one study, 42 young adults had blood tests that evaluated their immune function. Half were depressed, half were not. Compared with the normal participants, the depressed group showed significant immune impairment.[13]

- Depression can affect the dosing requirements of your medications. It can also put you at greater risk of experiencing side effects.

- Depression robs you of the mental stamina you need to live with a chronic illness. You are less able to take control of your disease and improve the quality of your life.

If you are feeling depressed, don't lump the symptoms with those of fibromyalgia. Depression is a highly treatable condition that you can do something about.

The Overlap Dilemma

Major depression makes it almost impossible to carry on usual activities, sleep, eat, or enjoy life. Pleasure seems a thing of the past. The

National Institute for Mental Health (NIMH) says that if you have experienced four or more of the following symptoms for more than 2 weeks, you are at risk for clinical depression and should have a physical and psychological evaluation by a medical physician:

- A persistent sad, anxious, or "empty" mood
- Loss of interest or pleasure in ordinary activities, including sex
- Sleep problems (insomnia, oversleeping, early-morning waking)
- Eating problems (loss of appetite or weight, weight gain)
- Difficulty concentrating, remembering, or making decisions
- Feelings of hopelessness or pessimism
- Feelings of guilt, worthlessness, or helplessness
- Thoughts of death or suicide; a suicide attempt
- Irritability
- Excessive crying
- Recurring aches and pains that don't respond to treatment[14]

These are the facts about depression as we know them today, but if you look over that list again, you'll see that some of the symptoms of depression overlap with those of fibromyalgia. That is exactly why the two are often confused. In fact, because of this overlap, many people with fibromyalgia are incorrectly told they have depression. A study by Carol S. Burckhardt, R.N., Ph.D., and colleagues out of the Oregon Health Sciences University, found that commonly used tests for depression, particularly the Beck Depression Inventory test, use markers (e.g., fatigue, sleep difficulties, and effort required to get things done) that are not measuring depression but rather typical fibromyalgia symptoms and consequences. Dr. Burckhardt notes that because of this overlap, "patients with fibromyalgia are likely to continue to be seen as having high rates of depression. Not only are stereotypes reinforced in this manner, but health care providers may

Learn More

Find out more about depression by contacting these organizations:

National Foundation for Depressive Illness
P.O. Box 2257
New York, NY 10116
(800) 239-1265
www.depression.org

National Mental Health Association
1021 Prince Street
Alexandria, VA 22314
(800) 969-6642
www.nmha.org

fail to provide comprehensive treatment that takes into account both physical and psychological factors."[15]

So here is the dilemma: While there definitely are people who have fibromyalgia and depression and absolutely need to find proper treatment for both conditions, many people with fibromyalgia are being incorrectly diagnosed with depression, which compounds the difficulty of finding proper care and treatment. For this reason, it is vital to find a physician who understands the difference between depression and fibromyalgia.

Fighting the Battle of Depression

Thirty-two-year-old Stacie has a long history of depression. "I was 6 years old the first time I remember seriously wanting to kill myself," she says. "And there is a long line of depression and mental illness in my family." When Stacie actually did try to kill herself at the age of 16, the desperation was put off to "typical teenage angst." Her dad didn't believe in depression and would not allow her to take medication or receive any kind of therapy, so the problem continued. But when she found herself as a single mom with two kids, the depression was more than she could handle, and she again tried several times to kill herself.

Finally, between the ages of 20 and 24, Stacie received medical help, medications, and even electroconvulsive therapy. But the outcome was sometimes worse than the problem; as Stacie says, "I became an overmedicated zombie." Then at age 24, Stacie took an overdose and found herself flat-lining in a hospital emergency room. "This was not a cry for help," insists Stacie. "I just wanted to end it." But this attempt did not end it, and Stacie went on, struggling once again to keep her head above the water line.

"When I was 28," Stacie remembers, "I was feeling just awful. I was so tired, and I had a terrible sore throat. I just couldn't function. But my doctor wouldn't listen. She insisted that I was tired because I was overweight and that I had body aches and sleep problems because I had a history of depression. Case closed." This wasn't an unusual reaction. Stacie had learned that having had depression compounded the difficulty of getting an accurate diagnosis of other medical problems. Repeatedly, Stacie found herself being treated like she was a hypochondriac.

Finally, a new team of young osteopathic doctors opened a practice in Stacie's area. With nothing to lose, Stacie went to them to see whether, just maybe, they'd listen. They quickly diagnosed mononucleosis. A few months later Stacey was diagnosed with fibromyalgia. "This doctor is a really good person," smiles Stacie. "He doesn't judge me by my depression. He looks at my other symptoms separately and sees that there is more to me than just depression." Stacie believes that this attitude alone has helped her better manage her depression because now she's not constantly spending so much energy trying to get someone to listen to her—to really listen without prejudging.

Having an understanding and helpful doctor has turned things around for Stacie. Now she wants to be in control of her own physical and mental health. "I don't want to be overmedicated anymore. I don't want to be treated like I don't know what's going on. I research everything and learn as much as I can about my illness so I can help myself," she says. At one point, Stacie took a class for mental health professionals so she could get more insight into her illness. She also joined an outpatient program that gave her the tools she needed to help herself. "I've gotten much better because I want to be better," insists Stacie. "I can't sit around waiting for someone else to do something for me. Every day I struggle with depression, but I also make myself keep going."

Stacie has noticed that, although they are separate illnesses, her depression and the symptoms of her fibromyalgia are connected in many ways. "When I have a bad day with one, I usually also have a bad day with the other. For instance, last week I went to a university pain center, and I was told, 'Here are some medications, but we can't do anything for you.' This news made me extremely depressed, and then I started feeling really bad fatigue and muscle pain from the fibromyalgia. One jump-starts the other."

> Stacie has noticed that, although they are separate illnesses, her depression and the symptoms of her fibromyalgia are connected in many ways.

This is just one recent example of why Stacie knows she has to think positive. "This is my best weapon against both the depression and the fibromyalgia. I have to keep telling myself that I'm fine. This isn't denial; it's just a step I have to take to make myself feel a little better. When something makes it too hard for me to feel positive, like that trip to the pain center, I start to lose hope, and then the fibromyalgia acts up. When I feel myself slipping into a really bad depression, I've trained myself to sit down every hour and think of one thing that I'm happy about or write it down if I'm feeling really bad. I might say, 'I'm really happy that I can breathe.' The next hour I say, 'I'm really happy that I have five little puppies in my house who give me a lot of love.' The next hour I say, 'I have two wonderful children for whom I am grateful.' The next hour, 'I'm extremely lucky to have a wonderful man like Bob in my life.' This is really hard to do because when I'm depressed I don't give a damn, but I force myself. I have to do something to help myself, especially when I don't feel like it."

Having fibromyalgia makes it that much more difficult for Stacie to keep an upbeat attitude. But still she works to keep going. "The pain in my back and legs is so bad that I walk with a cane," says Stacie. "I hurt so bad that I haven't been able to make a family meal in three months. But I still know that I have to think positively. There's no way I can deal with the problems of fibromyalgia if I let the depression take over. Everything gets worse as soon as you give up. I'm not saying people with fibromyalgia don't have the right to pull the covers over their head and stay in bed on a really bad day. But you can do that only for one day. After that, you have to get up and face the day instead of hiding. You have to at least go outside for even a minute or call a good friend and talk. The things I do to help me avoid depression are the same things that help me live with fibromyalgia. I just have to keep going and accept the life I have and make the best of it."

MIND-BODY THERAPY

Although the exact cause of fibromyalgia is unclear and the pain and other symptoms of FMS are not just "all in your head," there is also no doubt that the mind can either improve or worsen these very real symptoms and change the way you experience this condition. Leslie Bourne, Ph.D., director of the division of behavioral medicine at Fallon Clinic in Worcester, Massachusetts, has worked for many years teaching people with fibromyalgia how to use the mind-body connection to manage pain and depression. "We know that people's thoughts have a big impact on the body psychologically," says Dr. Bourne. "For example, if you're having negative thoughts like, 'I'll never get better,' or, 'This is ruining my life,' that will impact your ability to emotionally cope with the pain.

"But these thoughts can also work against you on a very physical level," she continues. "Negative thoughts begin a spiral of physical reactions that start in the brain and can lead to physical changes that can increase the experience of pain—sympathetic nervous system activity can release chemicals like adrenaline and the stress hormone cortisol; you can then experience physical changes such as rapid heart rate, muscle tension, and increased blood pressure, which can exacerbate your symptoms."

This reaction to negative thoughts sets off a pain cycle (see figure 5.1). The pain of fibromyalgia causes negative thoughts that trigger the body's stress response, that can cause more pain, causing more negative thoughts!

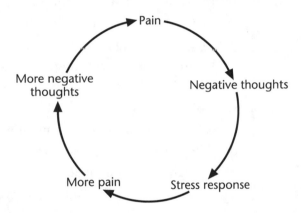

Figure 5.1—*Pain Cycle*

Fortunately, you can use the mind-body aspect of fibromyalgia to interrupt this pain cycle and have an impact on the central nervous system's perception of pain. Dr. Bourne says that because we know that the mind sends signals to all parts of the body that can set off a stress response exacerbating pain, it's critical to intervene at the point where this begins—at the level of thought. A mind-body therapy called cognitive/behavioral therapy is often used to do this. "Cognitive and behavioral strategies have been shown to be very effective for nonpharmacologic management of pain," Dr. Bourne says.

Cognitive-Behavioral Therapy

Cognitive-behavioral therapy (CBT) focuses on negative and noncoping thoughts and actions caused by persistent pain, repeated treatment failures, and the tendency of pain sufferers to focus their attention on their pain so intently that it comes to dominate their lives to the exclusion of other activities.

When obsession with pain allows it to become the controlling life force, a great sense of helplessness and hopelessness can result. Cognitive-behavioral therapy turns that helplessness around by giving you control. It teaches you that you are not a hapless victim. It shows you that the way you think about your illness, and therefore the way you act, can strongly influence the way you live with this chronic condition.

> *CBT shows you that the way you think about your illness, and therefore the way you act, can strongly influence the way you live with this chronic condi-*

Cognitive-behavioral therapy is best learned and practiced under the guidance and supervision of a trained therapist. Treatment may be provided on an inpatient or outpatient basis depending on your needs and the availability of such programs in your area.

Studies on CBT and fibromyalgia have shown very positive results. One particular study by Drs. Nielson, Walker, and McCain in 1992, reported favorable results among 25 fibromyalgia patients who participated in a 3-week, inpatient cognitive-behavioral therapy program. A follow-up study published in 1995 by Drs. White and Nielson found that 2 to 4 years after the completion of the first study, the 25 participants maintained the beneficial results in three areas: sense of control over the illness, degree of worry, and observed pain behavior. These results are especially impressive considering that FMS symptoms tend to worsen with time despite drug therapy.[16] Another study by Dr. Betsy B. Singh and colleagues out of the University of Maryland School of Medicine found CBT offered significant reduction in pain, fatigue, and sleeplessness and improved function, mood state, and general health following an 8-week program.[17]

In typical cognitive-behavioral therapy sessions, it's likely you will work on both cognitive and behavioral strategies at the same time, but for your own information, consider how each works to relieve pain and reduce the likelihood of depression.

Cognitive Therapy

Cognition is a word used to refer to a person's thinking, perception, and memory. For a person in chronic pain, the basis of cognitive therapy (developed by American psychologist Aaron Beck in the late 1960s) is this: People who think they can control their pain, who avoid thinking the worst about their condition, and who believe they are not severely disabled appear to function better than those who do not. Cognitive therapy can be extremely effective in treating the emotional distress that results from the effects of chronic pain.

To begin therapy, you are asked to keep track of how you think about your pain, with a view to ban negative self-talk such as this:

> *People who think they can control their pain, who avoid thinking the worst about their condition, and who believe they are not severely disabled appear to function better than those who do not.*

- **Do you catastrophize?**

  "This is the worst pain in the world."
  "My life is ruined."

- **Do you overgeneralize?**

  "No one understands me."
  "This will never end."

- **Do you personalize?**

  "Leave it to me to have this kind of pain."
  "I guess I deserve to live like this."

- **Do you obsess?**

  "This is awful. This is terrible. I can't stand this."

When you find yourself thinking these kinds of negative thoughts, ask yourself:

- **"How does this thought affect my mood?"**
  (It probably pulls it down immediately.)

- **"How does this thought affect me physically?"**
  (You probably tighten up and feel more pain.)

These thoughts are not wrong or bad. Who could have chronic pain or depression and not have these thoughts? But they make a bad situation worse. Fortunately, they are one part of your life that you can take control of to improve your medical state. This is done through a process called *cognitive restructuring*—changing the way you think about your illness. This is much more than just positive thinking. Saying to yourself, "This isn't so bad," probably won't make you feel any better, but you can change the way your body physically responds if you retrain your mind to challenge negative thoughts.

> *Y*ou can change the way your body physically responds if you retrain your mind to challenge negative thoughts.

There are many different styles of restructuring a therapist might choose to teach you. A typical example is one that asks you to interrupt the negative thought, examine it for truth, and then find another way to think about the situation that gives you some control. The following two examples will give you an idea of how this works.

Example 1

Let's say you feel just awful after taking a 20-minute walk and can't get back on your feet for the rest of the day. You say to yourself, "I always feel worse after I exercise. What's the point? It's no use even trying to exercise."

Immediately begin cognitive restructuring:

Step 1—Interrupt: "Stop. Don't go any further with this negative thought."

Step 2—Examine: "Do I really *always* feel worse after exercise? Will I really feel better if I give up exercise completely?"

Step 3—Take control: "I shouldn't walk for 20 minutes. Next time I'll cut it down to 10 minutes and see how I feel."

Example 2

Let's say you're having a bad flare and hear yourself say, "Why does this always happen at the worst possible time?!" Immediately begin cognitive restructuring:

Step 1—Interrupt: "Wait a minute. Don't go any further with this negative thought."

Step 2—Examine: "Does *every* flare I have *always* happen at the worst time?" Then think of flares you've had that came on during very typical, common periods of time when nothing special was going on.

Step 3—Take control: "This flare has come at a very bad time. But I'm not going to push myself too hard and make things worse. Maybe this won't last too long, and I'll eventually get done all the things I need to do. I'll get through this one day at a time just like I've done in the past." This gives you a different way of looking at the situation.

You can also use kind affirmations to restructure the way you talk to yourself. Instead of kicking yourself and saying things like, "I'm so pathetic," or, "How could anybody love me?" be kind to yourself with loving words. Make a habit of saying things like the following:

- It takes a courageous person to live with this illness.
- I love and believe in myself.
- I'm learning how to take control of this illness and live a good life.
- I accept myself the way I am and will make the best of this life I have.
- I am a good person.

Cognitive therapy will help you recognize your own self-talk attitudes and identify the negative statements you say to yourself that are making it harder for you to live with a chronic condition. As a person living with fibromyalgia, it's vital to your disease management that you understand the clear relationship between the way you think about your health and the way you feel it.

Behavioral Therapy

Behavioral therapists believe that all behavior is learned and that certain learned behaviors can get you stuck in the pain cycle and actually promote and aggravate your illness. Behavior modification is designed to break negative behavior patterns such as drug taking, avoidance of activity, dependence on others, and preoccupation with pain. This therapy encourages and rewards the very opposite of these behaviors: responsibility, independence, activity, and the desire to free oneself from pain rather than be bound to it.

Leslie Nadler, Ph.D., who is a psychologist and director of behavioral therapy at Pain Care in Long Island, New York, believes that the first goal in behavior modification is to identify the triggers that prompt what he calls "negative pain behaviors." "A pain trigger can be almost anything. It can even be certain people in your life, for example. Consider the young child who falls down in the playground. If his

Effective Treatment

The most effective treatment program for fibromyalgia includes:

- Medication for pain and fatigue
- Gentle daily exercise
- Relaxation strategies
- Cognitive-behavioral therapy

mom is nearby, it's likely he'll howl with pain. If she is not, although the pain is still very real, he may choose to pick himself up and run back to play. This same pain behavior happens in our own households.

"A trigger can also be boredom," he continues. "A trigger might be a high state of emotional anxiety. There is an endless possibility of pain triggers. I recently worked with a woman who had fibromyalgia and was surprised to find that her pain was triggered by the time of day; at 2:30 P.M. just before her children came home from school, her pain levels increased. The anticipation of the stress of running her kids from place to place after school made her muscles tense, the blood flow decreased to that area, and her pain increased. I've seen other people whose pain would increase when they subconsciously anticipated the moment that the effects of their pain medication were about to wear off. These are all triggers that affect the way we feel pain."

These triggers elicit behavioral consequences. It might be a verbal complaint like, "Oh, my aching back." Or it may be the decision to stay home from work. Or you may reach for more medication. Or the trigger may signal that it's time to get back into bed and wait for the pain or fatigue to ease. Dr. Nadler warns, "If the consequences of these behaviors are positive, the behavior will increase. If, for example, you get attention when you complain, you'll continue to complain. If you can avoid doing an unpleasant task because you are in pain, you might find yourself more aware of your pain."

A behavioral therapist will help you examine all the triggers and consequences that surround your pain and fatigue. He or she may ask you to ask yourself questions like these:

- Do I avoid physical activity to "protect" myself?
- Have I stopped socializing because of my illness?
- Do I want others to take care of me?
- Do I rely on medication to control my illness?
- Do I often groan, limp, rub, brace myself, or talk about my illness and pain?

- Do I get attention by talking about my illness?

- Do I use my illness to avoid undesirable activities?

- Do I sustain my illness in the hope of gaining monetary compensation?

Some people become defensive when a therapist asks them to think about these types of behaviors, but the questions are not insulting—they simply require an honest reevaluation of how you may be reacting to a very difficult chronic illness. Dr. Nadler continues:

I never want a patient to think I'm suggesting that the pain isn't real. You have a physical illness that has a physical base to it, but still you may develop pain behaviors based on the way you think about and react to your pain. Identifying these behaviors will not get rid of your pain—behavioral therapy does not focus on the pain but rather on the pain behaviors. The goal is to modify some of the behaviors that are frequently associated with pain.

It's interesting, however, that when they modify those behaviors, often people find that they do indeed feel less pain. It's really not that the pain has gone away but that the level of suffering has gone down. People begin to realize that the way they react to their pain and fatigue can be reinforced in a positive or a negative way. They can learn to do things that reduce the way their illness or condition negatively influences their quality of life.

This is not to say that they don't have real pain and fatigue. These symptoms of fibromyalgia are very real—but you have a choice about how you react to them. I say to my patients, "You have real pain, but would you agree that there are many different ways you can express that pain? There are probably some ways that are good ways to express pain and other ways that are less helpful. Let's look at your pain behaviors." We're not talking about the pain itself but rather how a person expresses it.

> *B*ehavioral therapy does not focus on the pain but rather on the pain behaviors. The goal is to modify some of the behaviors that are frequently associated with pain.
>
> —LESLIE NADLER, PH.D.

After the pain triggers and consequences have been identified, it's time to develop pain behavior patterns that are more positive and helpful. You will begin to do things that shift your focus from your pain to other aspects of your life. A sampling of the strategies Dr. Nadler uses include pacing, scheduled fun, pleasurable activities, sleep hygiene, and realistic goal setting.

Pacing

This strategy asks you to pace yourself—find a balance. Rather than go into overdrive on the days you feel good and end up unable to move for the next 2 days, find a comfortable level of activity and stick to that level both when you feel great and when you feel not so great. You'll find you can do more if you do a little bit consistently than if you push to do a great amount and then face the consequence of extended downtime.

Dr. Nadler believes that when pacing, it's best not to use your pain as a guideline of when to stop. "I think it's better to pace based on activity levels rather than pain level. For example, if you know you can walk two blocks without great pain, fatigue, or physical risk, do that. Even if you feel great and want to go farther, stop at two blocks. If you're having a bad day, do the two blocks anyway because you know you can do it. If you know you can ride the exercise bike for 3 minutes, stop there even when you're feeling great, and push to 3 minutes even when you're feeling poorly. Some doctors tell patients to stop when it hurts, but if you do that you'll never get anywhere. It will be very hard to make progress because there is such variability. One day you'll be doing a lot and the next day you'll be doing nothing. I recommend doing a moderate amount on a consistent basis."

Scheduled Fun

You need to have a life outside your disease. You may have already given up a lot because of the daily pain and fatigue, but you cannot give up finding joy in life. You may often not feel like having fun or socializing, but if you can push yourself to do this, you'll start to feel better more often. It's kind of like saying, "You will have fun whether you like it or not," but it works.

Look at your calendar and schedule in some fun time. Plan to call an old friend and chat. Plan to put your feet up and read a book or take a long bath. Plan to meet a friend for dinner. You may not be up to a ski weekend, but there are certainly some things you can do and enjoy. Write them on your calendar and do them!

> *Y*ou may have already given up a lot because of the daily pain and fatigue, but you cannot give up finding joy in life.

Pleasurable Activities

Because of your pain and fatigue, have you given up activities that you previously enjoyed doing? Choose one or two of those activities, and plan to give them another try. But before doing this, Dr. Nadler asks his patients to record a prediction beforehand on a scale of 0 to 10 of two things:

1. How effectively they will do it.

2. How much pleasure they will get out of doing it.

"My experience is that people usually make predictions from a very negative mind-set and set very low-level predictions," he explains. "But then they often find that in reality things are better than they thought they would be. It's not a matter of having as much pleasure or mastery as previously but of finding that these things can still be a source of pleasure."

Sleep Hygiene

Knowing sleep issues often are a part of fibromyalgia, Dr. Nadler emphasizes sleep behaviors in his therapy sessions. He believes that you can do a number of things to improve the quality of your sleep, including these:

- If you're not able to fall asleep within a half hour, get up. Don't lie in bed thinking about how you can't sleep.

- Make sure you go to bed around the same time each evening to normalize your sleep patterns.

- Get up in the morning at the same time each day. It is counterproductive to stay in bed longer to try to make up for lost hours during the night.

- Don't do anything that is overly stimulating, such as exercising, too close to sleep time.

- Take a warm bath or drink a glass of warm milk before bedtime.

Realistic Goal Setting

The fastest way to defeat yourself and fall back into the "I can't" mind-set is to set goals that are too ambitious. If, with the best intentions, you decide to squeeze into your hectic day 1 hour of relaxation exercises, a half hour of exercise, and a leisurely phone chat with a good friend, you're bound to fail. Although all these things would be good for you, it's unlikely that you can do them every day without feeling the incredible stress that comes with unrealistic overscheduling. Set reachable, small goals, and increase them as you're able.

If you're new to self-help activities, 5 minutes of relaxation exercises every other day with 5 minutes of gentle stretching exercise on the off days is a great place to start. If you want to ride a stationary bike, ride for a minute or two and stop while you still feel good. Don't push and overdo it and end up in pain; this will teach you that exercise is painful.

Cognitive-behavioral therapy definitely belongs in your treatment program for FMS. If you are not under the care of a trained therapist, don't dismiss the idea of CBT completely. You can do many of these mind-body strategies on your own. With some persistence and practice, you can learn to identify your negative thoughts and behaviors, challenge them, and replace them with more appropriate thoughts and actions. When you learn to change the way you think about your pain (cognitive therapy) and the way you act in response to your pain (behavioral therapy), you have a powerful mind-body tool that will give you back a good life. It may not be the same life you had before fibromyalgia, but it can be a good one with lots of hope for a fulfilling future.

Finding Balance

Emily is a 26-year-old logistics analyst and assistant project manager. She was diagnosed with fibromyalgia 4 years ago after she suffered severe nausea "that hit like a ton of bricks" followed by extreme exhaustion. Emily can't point to a particular trigger that brought on this illness; she was taking classes to earn her second bachelor's degree and found that after the subway ride to her classes she was just too sick and tired to do anything once she got there. Fortunately, Emily was already under the care of a rheumatologist because she has rheumatoid arthritis as well—which actually made things more confusing at first because as Emily says, "I just hurt all over—it's hard to tell one from the other sometimes." Although it's been a game of HMO roulette, Emily feels she's been very lucky to have good doctors. "Even my primary care doctor was able to see that something else besides arthritis and depression was going on even though there were no test results pointing to anything specific."

> *When you learn to change the way you think about your pain (cognitive therapy) and the way you act in response to your pain (behavioral therapy), you have a powerful mind-body tool that will give you back a good life.*

In addition, Emily has had bipolar disorder "all" her life. She says, "I was diagnosed with this problem when I was 20, but I've had the symptoms for as long as I can remember." Given this long history, certainly Emily's depressive episodes are not the cause or the result of fibromyalgia. In fact, in Emily's case, the conditions seem to be quite separate. "I'd have to say that my depressive episodes don't really affect my fibromyalgia, and my fibromyalgia flares don't seem to trigger depression. But some things about fibromyalgia (like the times when I

> ## Spiritual Strength
>
> John Astin, Ph.D., researcher and assistant professor at the University of Maryland School of Medicine in the Complementary Medicine Program, believes that "the challenge is to find inner strength to carry on in the face of chronic pain. Spiritual faith can certainly be a source of that strength. How that happens is questionable, but feeling a connection to something larger than oneself may provide a perspective within which physical pain is more manageable because it's not all-consuming. Spirituality can supply the joy and hope that is often missing in lives touched by chronic illness."

just can't think straight enough to read the back of a cereal box) do make me feel very frustrated, and I know I have to do something positive to keep everything from going downhill fast."

Emily says she learned very early on to deal quickly with stressful things that could bring on depression. "I'm careful to take medication when I need it. I look for the support of my friends and family who keep me going when things are really bad. (If I didn't have their support, I'd be toast by now!) And I also talk to myself a lot to keep myself from sinking. I remind myself that this will pass. I try to focus on the promise of an upswing.

"I also have adjusted my life so I can be more patient with myself and do what I can and not stress about everything else. If I can get something done—good. If I can't, there's no point stressing about it because that will just make the flare worse. I don't want to sit at home on my buns and eat bon-bons all day, but I also can't push myself so hard that I end up with a bad flare. I have to find a balance between rest and activity. Sometimes my activity level can be very high; sometimes it's low, and I'll take sick leave so I can work fewer hours. I think patience is the key to living with a chronic illness."

With large doses of patience, Emily seems to have found the balance that she looks for. Her significant other gives support and understanding; her job and her 18-month-old daughter keep her moving even when she doesn't feel like it. And her own determination not to give up keeps her spirits up and gives her hope.

THE MOST IMPORTANT GIFT

Stefan Kuprowski, N.D., director of the Ecomed Wellness Clinic in British Columbia, Canada, treats many FMS patients. "FMS requires people to take responsibility for their own healing," he believes, "to seek the right professional help and therapies, and transform their attitude toward the illness from curse to an incredible opportunity for growth and self-transformation. No small task, but that is what is required to heal." He says that because there are multiple causes to this illness, there are multiple cures. "What works for one person may not work for another due to biochemical individuality. Do not give up; the most important gift is the power of faith in the healing process and faith in oneself to heal."[18]

> *Hope is very important to how you experience this illness.*

Keep these words in mind when you feel that having fibromyalgia is like falling into a pit with no way out. And remember that those who are strong advocates for the recognition of fibromyalgia as a disease based in a physiological dysfunction believe that there are many things you can do to improve your daily functioning and quality of life. Although we still don't know a lot about fibromyalgia, we do know what helps people and improves their lives. Hope is very important to how you experience this illness.

In this multifaceted approach to fibromyalgia, we have looked at the treatment standards that include medication, exercise, relaxation, and mind-body awareness. Now the next chapter will explore the many options in complementary and alternative treatment therapies.

CHAPTER 6

Complementary and Alternative Therapies

B ECAUSE CONVENTIONAL MEDICINE doesn't have all the answers, many people with fibromyalgia turn to complementary and alternative medicine (CAM). In fact, researchers from Boston conducted a telephone survey of 20 people with fibromyalgia and found that within the past year, 100 percent had used at least one CAM therapy.[1] No one type of CAM has risen above the others as the "cure" for fibromyalgia, but many have offered relief and hope. The CAM therapies commonly used by people with fibromyalgia and discussed in this chapter add to your list of treatment options that give you some control over how you manage your illness. They include acupuncture, chiropractic, guaifenesin, herbs and supplements, homeopathy, massage, and nutrition.

A combination of both scientific research and anecdotal evidence shows that these therapies have helped some people with fibromyalgia reach the goals of improving the quality of sleep, reducing pain, increasing neurotransmitter production, and ultimately regaining control of physical and emotional health. This is not an all-inclusive list—there are other therapies out there you might want to try. Those discussed in this chapter will give you a place to start.

Alternative Choices

A telephone survey of 20 people with fibromyalgia found that at least 50 percent used nutritional supplements, relaxation, prayer, meditation, or massage therapy, and 25 to 40 percent used imagery, chiropractic, herbal therapies, yoga, acupuncture, or topical therapies. They spent between $70 and $3,767. The most costly were chiropractic ($792 per year), massage therapy ($773 per year), and acupuncture ($412 per year). The therapies most commonly thought to be effective at treating FMS symptoms were relaxation, imagery, and acupuncture.[2]

PLOT YOUR PROGRESS

When you use CAM therapies to treat the various symptoms of fibromyalgia, take it slowly. If you jump in with both feet and try many approaches at the same time, you'll have no way of knowing what is working and what is not. In the article "Using Alternative Treatments," Pat Randolph, director of psychological services at Texas Tech Medical Center's pain clinic, advises, "If you're thinking of trying more than one type of alternative therapy for your condition, don't try them all at once. Evaluate one first, then another, either alone or combined with the first (if your doctor agrees that the combination is safe)."[3]

A good way to do this evaluation is to plot your progress carefully. Ask your practitioner whether there are objective ways to measure improvement in your condition. If so, have any necessary tests or measurements taken before starting the treatment you've chosen. Also, note how bad your symptoms are, using a scale of 0 (no symptoms) to 10 (unbearable). During treatment, keep a daily symptom diary, again using the 0 to 10 scale and adding any specific details that seem important. After a month or two, review your symptom diary with your doctor and have any necessary tests or measurements done to assess your progress. This should give you a good idea of whether you're getting any real benefit from the treatment.

COMPLEMENTARY AND ALTERNATIVE THERAPIES

Many legitimate and effective complementary and alternative therapies are available to treat fibromyalgia. There are also many that teeter on the edge between legitimate and unproven that await further study. And, of course, many also are no more than fraudulent quackery. The following therapies are those that many physicians, natural healers, and people with fibromyalgia agree often have a positive effect on the symptoms of fibromyalgia.

What to Ask

Before you begin any CAM therapy, ask the practitioner these questions:

- Does the therapy you use help people with fibromyalgia? What evidence do you have?

- Have you treated patients with fibromyalgia? May I talk to them?

- How much will this therapy cost, and how many visits will be necessary before we know whether it's working?

- Could this therapy interfere with my conventional care?

- Are you willing to discuss your plans with my medical doctor?

If you decide to give complementary and alternative medicine a try, you'll need to do a bit of investigating first. In each case, the system of licensing practitioners varies from state to state; to find a trained and competent therapist, you should contact the national organization listed in each section for a sound referral. The fees for these services also vary from one practitioner to another, and insurance coverage is never a sure thing. Some insurance companies will cover CAM therapies, others cover it in certain circumstances, and still others will not touch it. Find out how much this will cost you before you jump in.

Acupuncture

Acupuncture is one of the major Asian healing arts that involves the use of fine needles inserted at specific points on the body. This therapy originated in China thousands of years ago and is based on the theory that an essential life energy called *qi* (pronounced "chee") flows through the body along invisible channels called meridians. When the flow of qi is blocked or is out of balance, illness or pain results. It is believed that stimulation of specific points along the meridians can correct the flow of qi to restore or optimize health or to block pain.

> *Many conventional doctors do not believe in the existence of qi, but few argue with the scientific research that supports the use of acupuncture.*

Many conventional doctors do not believe in the existence of qi, but few argue with the scientific research that supports the use of acupuncture as an adjunctive therapy in the treatment of fibromyalgia. A 1999 study out of Sweden reported results typical of many of these studies. These investigators analyzed the short- and long-term effects on pain and other fibromyalgia symptoms of traditional Chinese acupuncture. Participants were nine 24- to 62-year-old patients who received acupuncture in 10 to 14 sessions over 2 to 3 months, followed by a 6-month observation period. Patients were evaluated at 4, 8, 12, and 24 weeks. Pain, sleep, medication, muscle tension, psychological tension, general well-being, number of tender points, and range of movement in shoulders and neck were assessed. In general, significantly greater changes occurred during the acupuncture than during the medical management period. The number of tender points was significantly decreased, and sense of well-being significantly improved up to 12 weeks. A significant decrease in general pain persisted for 8 weeks. Muscle tension and local pain in head, neck, and shoulder were significantly reduced throughout the 24-week period.[4] Results like these are hard to argue with.

In an interview for the *Fibromyalgia Network* newsletter, Miles Belgrade, M.D., a neurologist and acupuncturist from Minneapolis, Minnesota, explained: "Acupuncture should no longer be considered in the category of snake oil or voodoo. Unlike many other alternative medicines, acupuncture does have a scientific foundation. It's a foundation that is consistent with the Western scientific thinking in pain medicine biology. The evolution of our understanding of endorphins—the pain-fighting chemicals produced by the body—has helped acupuncture move forward in its scientific basis."[5]

The scientific explanation for the success of acupuncture is that needling the acupuncture points stimulates the nervous system to release endorphins. Indeed, researchers can measure an increase in endorphins in the spinal fluid of pain patients receiving acupuncture. The process can also trigger the release of other chemicals and hormones that influence the body's own internal regulating system. These include serotonin, norepinephrine, and substance P (the three neurotransmitters that happen to be out of balance in people with FMS).

> *Acupuncture should no longer be considered in the category of snake oil or voodoo. Unlike many other alternative medicines, acupuncture does have a scientific foundation.*
>
> —MILES BELGRADE, M.D.

Whether its power is due to the movement of qi or the release of neurotransmitters, acupuncture is gaining ground as a recognized treatment for fibromyalgia. In 1997, the National Institutes of Health (NIH) convened a consensus panel to provide a responsible assessment of the use and effectiveness of acupuncture to treat a variety of conditions. The panel concluded that there is sufficient evidence to support the use of acupuncture as the primary therapy in adult postoperative and chemotherapy nausea and vomiting and in postoperative dental pain. Painful conditions in which the NIH felt acupuncture may prove to be a promising add-on therapy include fibromyalgia, headache, menstrual cramps, myofascial pain, osteoarthritis, low back pain, and carpal tunnel syndrome.[6]

Barbara Gilbertson, D.O., board member of the American Academy of Medical Acupuncture and the medical director of the Klamath Pain Clinic in Klamath Falls, Oregon, agrees that acupuncture can be a valuable therapy for people with fibromyalgia. "Acupuncture addresses many of the related problems of fibromyalgia," she says. "One of the first things I want to do when I see a new patient with fibromyalgia is treat the problem with insomnia, which acupuncture can do very effectively. There are also certain regional points that allow acupuncture to promote muscle relaxation. And rather than use medication injections into trigger points, I find needling is much less traumatic, and I like the results better. Acupuncture can also relieve the problems caused by the overlapping conditions such as migraines, irritable bowel syndrome, and arthritis in a large percentage of people."

But acupuncture alone is usually not a magic cure. Dr. Gilbertson believes her patients who get the most benefit from acupuncture are those who use other therapies as well. "Those who also use exercise, cognitive-behavioral therapy, and stress reduction techniques seem to respond best to acupuncture."

Using Acupuncture

Everyone who considers using acupuncture wants to know, "Does it hurt?" The American Academy of Medical Acupuncture says that people experience medical acupuncture needling differently, but most people feel only minimal sensation as the needles are inserted; some feel nothing at all. No pain is felt once the needles are properly in place. Because acupuncture needles are very thin and solid and their points are smooth, as opposed to hollow needles with cutting edges like hypodermic needles, insertion through the skin is not as painful as injections or blood sampling.

The number of treatments needed differs from person to person. For a complex and chronic problem like fibromyalgia, eight to ten treatments over 1 to 2 months is an appropriate trial.[7]

Acupuncture is generally safe, but as with any therapy, you should be cautious. Judith Horstman, author of *The Arthritis Foundation's Guide to Alternative Therapies*, offers the following advice if you decide to use acupuncture to treat the symptoms of fibromyalgia:

> *Most people feel only minimal sensation as the needles are inserted; some feel nothing at all. No pain is felt once the needles are properly in place.*

- Get a diagnosis from a medical doctor before undergoing acupuncture to make sure you don't have a condition requiring prompt medical attention.

- Don't stop your medications without consulting your doctor. Acupuncture works with, not instead of, conventional medicine.

- Tell the acupuncturist about all health conditions, including pregnancy, and list all medications (including herbs and nonsteroidal anti-inflammatory drugs, which could cause you to bleed).

- Be sure the acupuncturist uses sterilized or disposable needles.

- Don't take muscle relaxants, tranquilizers, or painkillers right before acupuncture because acupuncture can intensify the effects of these drugs.

- Tell the practitioner right away if you experience pain. Acupuncture shouldn't hurt after the initial sting of the needle's insertion.

Referral Resources

To find a list of accredited acupuncturists, contact the following organizations:

National Certification Commission for Acupuncture and Oriental Medicine
Phone: (703) 548-9004
E-mail: info@nccaom.org
Web site: www.nccaom.org

American Academy of Medical Acupuncture
This organization offers a list of medical doctors and osteopathic physicians.
Phone: (800) 521-2262
Web site: www.medicalacupuncture.org

- Do not automatically take herbs offered by traditional Chinese practitioners. They can interact with prescription drugs.

- Track your progress. If you have no response at all after four to six sessions, this therapy may not work for you. Or you may want to try another therapist because, as in any therapy, skill levels vary.[8]

Chiropractic

The word *chiropractic* means "treatment by the hands, or manipulation." It is a system of healing that was developed by David Daniel Palmer in 1895. Palmer believed that displacements of the spine caused pressure on nerves, which created pain or symptoms in other parts of the body. Chiropractic treatment and patient management include a variety of procedures used in accordance with the treating doctor's education, experience, and best clinical judgment. These include (but are not limited to) chiropractic adjustments, manipulation, mobilization, physiotherapeutic modalities and procedures, exercise rehabilitation, nutritional counseling, ergonomics advice, and supportive appliances. Chiropractors use x rays and orthopedic and neurological tests in the diagnostic process.

A chiropractic treatment, which is drug-free and nonsurgical, often focuses on adjustment and manipulation. *Adjustments* involve dynamic thrusts (rapid, precise, and painless force) to a specific vertebra to remove any interference with nerves. *Manipulations* are more general reorderings of bones to realign joints and increase a person's range of motion.[9]

Studies have found that therapeutic manipulation has a role in the management of fibromyalgia. One study included 15 adult members of a regional fibromyalgia association who received chiropractic treatments, including ischemic compression and spinal manipulation.

> *A chiropractic treatment, which is drug-free and nonsurgical, often focuses on adjustment and manipulation.*

The researchers found that 30 treatments reduced the intensity of the participants' pain, sleep disturbance, and fatigue. They also found that the improvement in all three measures was maintained after 1 month without treatment.[10] In another earlier study, researchers gave 21 fibromyalgia patients (ages 25 to 70 years) treatment consisting of 4 weeks of spinal manipulation, soft tissue therapy, and passive stretching. The study reported that this chiropractic management improved patients' cervical and lumbar ranges of motion, straight-leg raise, and reported pain levels.[11]

Urscia Mahring, D.C., a member of the American Chiropractic Association, who is in practice in Alexandria, Virginia, has treated fibromyalgia patients for 15 years. Dr. Mahring feels that chiropractic care offers effective management of the symptoms of fibromyalgia. She strongly encourages people with this illness to use chiropractic therapy to better enable them to participate fully in the activities of daily life and in a wide range of exercise programs. "One of the very positive things about chiropractic in the treatment of fibromyalgia," says Dr. Mahring, "is that it can help reduce pain enough so a person can begin and continue an active exercise program, despite the inevitable symptom flare-ups experienced with exercise. Exercise is the best long-term self-management tool for fibromyalgia sufferers."

Dr. Mahring also feels that people with fibromyalgia may find particular benefit in the ability of chiropractic care to improve nervous-system functioning. Nerve interference can promote sickness and disease when the vertebrae are misaligned or lacking in normal movement; the flow of messages from the brain to all the other cells in the body is distorted. This type of nerve interference creates disorganization of bodily processes that can cause or aggravate many of the symptoms of fibromyalgia.

It is important to choose an experienced chiropractic doctor through a medical or personal recommendation because chiropractic treatment involves highly specific adjustment of the spinal tissues. Always be certain that your chiropractor is state licensed and reputable. Never allow a "paraprofessional" or other unlicensed person to attempt a spinal manipulation; this could worsen your problem rather than help it.

> *Nerve interference can promote sickness and disease when the vertebrae are misaligned or lacking in normal movement; the flow of messages from the brain to all the other cells in the body is distorted.*

Upper Cervical Chiropractic Care

More than 250 different chiropractic procedures are in use today. If you try one procedure with one chiropractor and it doesn't improve your symptoms, don't write off this form of health care completely. You might find better results with another practitioner and another procedure. One particular kind of chiropractic work that has been shown to offer remarkable results to some people with fibromyalgia is called *upper cervical adjusting*.

Upper cervical adjusting is a chiropractic procedure (practiced by fewer than 2,000 chiropractors worldwide) that corrects the position of the top two vertebrae of the spine, the atlas, C1, and axis, C2. By correcting the tilt, shift, or rotation of these vertebrae, the effects of many conditions can be minimized or eliminated altogether. In addition to its positive effect on fibromyalgia, this procedure has also been helpful in the treatment of such diverse conditions as migraines; epilepsy; attention deficit disorder; hypertension; trigeminal neuralgia; TMJ; some forms of arthritis and carpal tunnel; immune system disorders; herniated disks; numbness and tingling in the limbs; allergies and asthma; neck, back, arm, and feet pain; sciatica; and more.

> ### Referral Resource
> You can get a referral to a trained chiropractor in your area by contacting:
>
> **American Chiropractic Association**
> 1701 Clarendon Boulevard
> Arlington, VA 22209
> Phone: (800) 986-4636
> Web site: www.amerchiro .org

The rational for these results is really quite simple. As your spinal cord comes out of your brain and brain stem it passes through the center of the C1 or atlas vertebra, which is the donut-shaped bone your skull sits on. Your spinal cord at that point consists of trillions of nerve fibers that "bottle-neck" through the small opening in the atlas. These fibers eventually branch off, carrying information to every part of your body. If the C1 is out of its proper positions it can irritate, constrict, or disrupt vital nerve signals to any portion of your body. This can cause muscle or joint pain, organ dysfunction, weakened immune system, and countless other conditions that you would not ordinarily relate to a problem originating in your neck.

Upper cervical vertebrae can become misaligned in many ways—for example, as a result of an accident, emotional trauma, or chemical toxicity in the body. Childbirth itself can move the atlas out of position because of the massive amounts of pressure on the head and neck of the baby as it passes down the birth canal. Or childhood accidents such as falling from a tree, bike, or skates can misalign it. In adulthood, the atlas can be shoved out of position during minor or major accidents such as sporting accidents, automobile accidents, or slips and falls. Some of the worst cases of atlas misalignment and resulting pain have been caused by minor car accidents such as being rear-ended.

If an upper cervical chiropractor finds, after an extensive x-ray analysis, that your atlas or axis are out of alignment, he or she will begin this corrective procedure. The repositioning of the atlas verte-bra is done by hand or by instrument. De-pending on the doctor's technique, it feels like a light tap, a brisk thrust, or a soft massage at the side of the neck as the atlas is moved precisely back into its correct position. The procedure cures nothing. It simply restores body balance and brain-to-body communication so that or-gans, limbs, and tissues can resume normal func-tioning. The body can now self-heal.

> *B*y correcting the tilt, shift, or rotation of these vertebrae, the ef-fects of many conditions can be minimized or eliminated altogether.

An upper cervical correction is not a one-time thing. It often takes many adjustments to gain full symptom relief—exactly how many depends on your body. Some people can hold their correction for several months, even a year at a time. Others have to be cor-rected once or twice a week in the beginning, then once or twice a month. Everyone is different. The doctor's objective is to make as precise an upper cervical correction as possible. Then he or she will help you maintain the correction with as few treatments as possible so that you can live pain-free. Practitioners of this treatment believe that, just like dental checkups and physicals, periodic upper cervical checkups should be part of your personal preventive health care program.

It's difficult to know whether your atlas or axis are misaligned without first having a thorough evaluation of your upper spine through x rays. But you can suspect this problem if you have one leg that is slightly shorter than the other. You may also notice that when you stand in front of a mirror one shoulder is slightly higher than the other and one hip is higher than the other. Another indication that your top vertebrae may be out of position is the occurrence of a variety of physical symptoms in your body that your medical doctor cannot explain through medical testing.

An Upper Cervical Success Story

The journey to find relief from her fatigue and pain has been a long one for Louella Harris. In 1958 at the age of 3, she contracted polio in Kenya, East Africa, exactly 8 months after she was given a polio vaccine. Then, 34 years later, she was diagnosed with postpolio syndrome and fibromyalgia.

Louella went through many conventional medical therapies throughout her life without relief—and for many years without explanation. "Although I was diagnosed with fibromyalgia only 8 years ago," says Louella, "I know that I've suffered from this illness all my life. I've always had trouble sleeping; I've had a weak immune system; I've had excruciating pain in the neck, shoulders, and elbows that eventually spread down into my legs. I've had chronic digestive problems with constipation and diarrhea since childhood. I had short-term memory loss and a major problem with fatigue."

When another round of testing in her early 20s showed no reason for her symptoms, Louella's internist announced that nothing was wrong with her physically. He pronounced that she was suffering from depression. "He was right," laughs Louella now. "I was so ill and so confused, of course I was depressed!"

> The procedure cures nothing. It simply restores body balance and brain-to-body communication so that organs, limbs, and tissues can resume normal functioning.

Louella left the doctor's office with painkillers and a recommendation that she exercise. But the pain grew so intense that Louella became confined to bed for months. Her husband, Richard, became her personal attendant. He dressed and fed her and helped with all her personal needs on a daily basis. Louella couldn't even sit up to watch television or hold a book. Then one day a friend gave her a piece of information that has changed her life.

Louella was told about the little-known chiropractic procedure called upper cervical adjustment that had been shown to help the symptoms of fibromyalgia. She quickly located one of the upper cervical chiropractors in her state and began her journey to wellness.

Referral Resource

For information or a referral to an upper cervical chiropractor, contact:

National Awareness Campaign for Upper Cervical Care, Inc.
Phone: (888) 622-8221
E-mail: infor@upper cervical.org
Web site: www.upper cervical.org

"This man turned out to be a highly skilled, big-hearted doctor who took the time to call me back and answer all my questions on the phone," remembers Louella. "He gave me no guarantees, but the information he shared with me gave me hope."

Four months after Louella first experienced precision upper cervical chiropractic, she was out of bed, back to work, and pregnant. Nine months later at the age of 39 she gave birth to a baby girl. Since that time she and her husband have founded the nonprofit organization National Awareness Campaign for Upper Cervical Care, Inc. Their goal is to bring attention and awareness to this procedure that has so dramatically improved the quality of Louella's life.

Guaifenesin

R. Paul St. Amand, M.D., is very familiar with fibromyalgia. He has it himself, as do his wife, his three daughters, and his nurse. This personal involvement with this complex illness has sent him on a search that has resulted in a unique treatment therapy that some people swear by and others disregard completely. It's one of those remedies you just have to try for yourself to see if it's best for you.

Dr. St. Amand believes that, like gout, which is caused by the kidney's inability to process and eliminate uric acid that then collects in the joints and causes swelling and pain, fibromyalgia is the result of a kidney defect that makes it difficult for the body to process phosphates. This causes the phosphates to build up on a cellular level, bind

Same Premise, Different Approach

Upper cervical chiropractic adjustments are based on the same theory of spinal cord compression popularized by the work of Dr. Michael Rosner of the University of Alabama in Birmingham and Dr. Dan S. Heffez of the Chicago Institute of Neurosurgery and Neuroresearch. These physicians found that some people with fibromyalgia have the same problem as those with Chiari syndrome and cervical spinal stenosis—a narrowing of the opening at the base of the skull or in the neck that compresses the lower part of the brain or spinal cord. These doctors believe that by surgically widening this area, symptoms will significantly improve (as discussed in chapter 1). Upper cervical chiropractors feel that cervical corrections are a safer and less invasive approach to the same problem.

with calcium, and stay in the blood. Excess phosphates in the blood cause fatigue, irritability, depression, and forgetfulness. When the concentration of phosphates in the blood becomes too high, the body dumps the phosphates into muscle cells, where they bind with calcium and become calcium phosphate. The presence of calcium phosphate signals the muscle to move causing constant activity day and night, year after year. Without rest, the muscle will eventually spasm and cause the pain. Through years of experimentation, Dr. St. Amand found that guaifenesin, an ingredient found commonly in cold preparations, helps the kidneys expel phosphate and relieve the symptoms of fibromyalgia.

Not everyone in the medical profession agrees with this theory—as Dr. St. Amand makes obvious in the title of his book, *What Your Doctor May Not Tell You About Fibromyalgia*. But a quick look at the history of guaifenesin shows that this medication, which is now used to loosen phlegm, may have some action that relieves muscle pain. "Back in 1530, in its original form, a tree bark extract called *guaiacum*, guaifenesin was in use for rheumatism," says Dr. St. Amand. "It was later also used to treat gout. A paper written in 1928 showed its value for easing growing pains and several other symptoms that now are not difficult to recognize as fibromyalgia. Guaiacum was later purified to guaiacolate and made its first appearance in cough mixtures about 70 years ago. Over 20 years ago it was synthesized and named *guaifenesin* and pressed into tablet form. Its original use, however, is not completely forgotten. In the new *Physician's Desk Reference for Herbal Medicines*, *Guaiacum officinale* is indicated for rheumatism."

> *S*ome believe that guaifenesin, an ingredient found commonly in cold preparations, helps the kidneys expel phosphate and relieve the symptoms of fibromyalgia.

Despite the debate over the ability of this "cough medicine" to treat the symptoms of fibromyalgia, Dr. St. Amand has many loyal followers. Those who attest to the value of guaifenesin in easing the symptoms of fibromyalgia are those who have had the determination to persist through the two difficult aspects of this treatment therapy: You'll get worse before you get better, and you have to rid your body of substances that contain salicylates.

When you use guaifenesin, you should be ready for the ups and downs of the reversal cycle. As guaifenesin cleans the body's cells, the excess phosphate is dumped into the bloodstream, which moves it to the kidneys. When the kidneys cannot process these large batches, the blood deposits minibatches throughout the body, causing widespread aches and pains. The symptoms of fibromyalgia appear to worsen until the kidneys catch up. This flare is often followed by a rest period during which you may feel "normal" for the first time in years, but then as the excess phosphates build up again, you may have another flare. This reversal cycle continues until the phosphates are cleared. This can be a difficult roller coaster ride of ups and downs, but it is evidence that the guaifenesin is working. Because it can be tricky finding the proper dosage, Dr. St. Amand recommends that you work with a medical physician when taking guaifenesin even though the drug is available over the counter.

Dr. St. Amand cautions that you must avoid salicylates because they block the action of guaifenesin and make the treatment completely ineffectual. Unfortunately, avoiding salicylates isn't easy. Salicylate is both a natural and synthetic substance that is found in common items like aspirin, facial cleansing creams, shampoos, conditioners, cosmetics, herbal remedies, muscle balms, toothpastes, deodorants, cough drops, suppositories, and many more products sold under countless trade names.

> *When you use guaifenesin, you should be ready for the ups and downs of the reversal cycle.*

Support for Guaifenesin

Using guaifenesin to treat the symptoms of fibromyalgia isn't easy—but it isn't easy having fibromyalgia, either. Many people who have persevered through the reversal cycle and have eliminated salicylates have found remarkable results. Aileen Goldberg is one of them.

Aileen leads a fibromyalgia support group of about 400 people in New York and Long Island and, based on her own experience, is very active in promoting the use of guaifenesin for the treatment of this puzzling syndrome. Aileen was hit with the symptoms of FMS during her first pregnancy in 1979, when her body chemistry seemed to change dramatically and lead her on a 20-year search for answers. At first, constant backaches that would come and go and then muscle pains in her back, arms, shoulders, legs, fingers, feet, toes, and neck began. About 10 years later Aileen started to have double and blurry vision.

"I figured that because I'm a CPA and use the computer a lot," Aileen says, "I was having some eye strain, and I could solve the problem by closing one eye. At this time I was up for partnership in my firm, working 70 hours a week, and as the eye pain increased, I thought maybe I should start slowing down and should see a doctor."

Unfortunately, the optometrist, ophthalmologist, and even neuro-ophthalmologist found nothing physically wrong with Aileen's eyes as her symptoms worsened to include unbearable eye pain. "At this point I was hoping the MRIs would show I had a brain tumor," recalls Aileen. "At least this would be something that could be cut out and give me a chance to live without pain."

Using guaifenesin to treat the symptoms of fibromyalgia isn't easy—but it isn't easy having fibromyalgia, either.

Finally, in 1995, a chronic facial pain specialist recognized that it was temporomandibular joint disorder (TMJ) that was causing the muscles in Aileen's face to spasm and cause the eye pain and vision problems. Then as he applied pressure to certain areas that seemed very sensitive, he asked, "Does your back also hurt? Your shoulders? Your neck? Do you have irritable bowel syndrome? Do you have mitral valve prolapse? Do you have trouble sleeping well? Do you feel very tired every day?" As Aileen answered yes to all these questions, the doctor said, "You also have fibromyalgia." The doctor explained that there was no known cause or cure for this disease and prescribed the antidepressant Elavil to help ease the symptoms. Over the next 2 years Aileen also tried, without success, Pamelor, Prozac, Neurontin, Flexeril, Klonopin, Norflex, Placquenil, Ambien, Restoril, methadone, morphine, Tylenol 3 with Codeine, Ultram, and many minerals, vitamins, amino acids, and supplements. All this while, Aileen was also receiving steroid injections twice a week to ease the muscle spasms in her face, neck, and shoulders. "I knew this couldn't be good for my body," says Aileen, "but at that point I didn't care what the long-term effects would be. Anything that improved my vision and eased my pain was fine with me."

One day in 1996, Aileen came across a book that mentioned the use of guaifenesin for the treatment of fibromyalgia. "Hey, I was ready to try anything," she recalls. "I was commuting to my job in New York City every day in terrible pain, and then I would sit at my desk and just cry. I had nothing to lose." Aileen found a complementary physician who did not know much about guaifenesin but was willing to prescribe it, knowing it had no known side effects and was a reasonable therapeutic attempt by someone in extreme, chronic pain who had tried everything else available.

A lot has happened since that day. Aileen feels she is now 90 percent better. She has visited Dr. St. Amand in California as a patient and has organized and hosted his presentations to medical practitioners and to people with fibromyalgia in New York City.

"If your doctor hasn't found anything else that helps you," Aileen suggests, "ask him to prescribe guaifenesin; if he doesn't want to, give him a copy of Dr. St. Amand's book. Learning something new about how to treat this terribly disabling condition would not be a bad thing. It's true that it can make you feel somewhat worse before you feel better, and you do have to use different makeup and body lotions to avoid salicylates, but I think it's worth it."

Aileen tells the members of her support group that they can take guaifenesin without giving up any of their other medications or therapies; it's just one more option to try. "I still see a psychotherapist because it's difficult living with chronic pain; I see a chiropractor who eases my trigger points; I've just begun working with an exercise trainer; I do cranial sacral therapy as a mind-body treatment; I still have massages; I practice meditation; and I've learned to slow my life down. Until I'm 100 percent cured, all these things help me live with fibromyalgia."

Herbs and Supplements

Kathleen Duffy, L.P.N., medical herbalist, certified clinical aromatherapist, and expert reviewer for the *Complete Guide to Natural Healing*, has worked with people with fibromyalgia since 1978, and she believes many natural supplements can relieve the symptoms. "But," cautions Duffy, "keep in mind that we're talking about treating a whole person—not just the symptoms. So what works best can vary from one person to another. Things like lifestyle, personality, and stress response will affect the way natural substances work in the body, so ideally, you will have a trained herbalist talk to you one-on-one to determine what is best for you individually."

> *What works best can vary from one person to another. Things like lifestyle, personality, and stress response will affect the way natural substances work in the body.*
>
> —KATHLEEN DUFFY, L.P.N.

Talking generally, Duffy usually recommends that the following herbs and supplements be taken daily to manage the symptoms of fibromyalgia:

- **B-complex supplement.** The B vitamins are good for promoting nerve strength, digestive functioning, and the ability to withstand the stresses of daily life (as well as the stress of chronic pain and poor sleep patterns). Take 100 milligrams daily with food.

- **Multivitamin with antioxidants.** This should include vitamins C, A, and E.

- **Digestive aid.** Betaine hydrochloride (HCL) and pepsin, apple cider vinegar, pancreatin, or bromelain support digestive juices and help the absorption of nutrients; they are also known for their anti-inflammatory properties.

- **Turmeric.** This yellow spice (*Curcuma longa*), often found in curry, can be used as an anti-inflammatory and antioxidant. Take one 300-microgram capsule two or three times a day. Some studies indicate that it may be as effective as cortisone without the side effects.

- **Powdered ginger.** This is a natural anti-inflammatory. Two 500-microgram capsules is the average dose, but those with an inflammatory condition may need to take more over a period of months. People with sensitive stomachs should take it with food.

- **Siberian ginseng.** This is an adaptogenic herb (*Eleutherococcus senticosus*) that will help you tolerate stress and nourish your glands. This also battles fatigue without putting a stimulant in your body. Take one or two 400-milligram capsules two or three times a day.

- **Skullcap.** This herb (*Scutellaria lateriflora*) is good for muscle pain and spasms. A cup of skullcap and spearmint tea is soothing, refreshing, and good tasting.

- **Boswellan cream.** *Boswella serratta*, a member of the frankincense family, was studied at the Government Medical College in Jammu, India, as a treatment for fibromyalgia and arthritis in the late 1980s. The results showed a 70 percent improvement in the pain response after topical application for 4 weeks.

- **Calcium and magnesium supplements.** Hair analysis has found that patients with fibromyalgia have significantly lower calcium and magnesium levels than those without fibromyalgia. Some fibromyalgia researchers believe that calcium and magnesium supplements can be an effective adjunctive therapy for fibromyalgia.[12] Twitches, leg cramps, and a craving for chocolate all indicate a possible lack of magnesium. Take 600 milligrams of calcium and 1,000 milligrams of magnesium daily. You can also try malic acid, 1,200 to 3,000 milligrams, on an empty stomach.

- **MSM (methyl sulfonyl methane).** This dietary form of sulfur improves enzyme production, helping the body create healthy cells. Take 1,000 milligrams daily.

To improve sleep, you might give Duffy's recommended essential oil bath and tea ritual a try. To prepare the bath, add two cups of Epsom salts to the bath water. (This gives your body a source of magnesium sulfate.) Then put some full-fat milk into a small glass (e.g., a shot glass), and add about 6 drops of an essential oil like true lavender, lavindin, or bergamot that contains esters and is extremely relaxing.

(Because oil and water don't mix, using milk allows the oil to disperse.) Add the milk-oil mixture to the bath. Soak up to your ears. If you don't have a tub or the time for a bath, do a foot soak for 20 minutes in the same solution (with only about 3 or 4 drops of the essential oil). Then try some chamomile, linden flower, valerian, or hops tea before bedtime. Each of these herbs has properties that help you unwind, relax, and sleep soundly.

Duffy does not recommend the supplement melatonin to her clients for their sleep problems. "It is a hormone," she explains, "and I have found that few people really have a melatonin deficiency, and so this has an extremely limited usefulness. I'd rather recommend an herbal or nutritional supplement and an alteration of lifestyle that I know will work and stay away from the 'pill-popping' mentality."

> *It is very important to work with your medical doctor when taking herbs along with other prescribed medications.*

It is very important to work with your medical doctor when taking herbs along with other prescribed medications. Currently no national system is in place for tracking which herb-drug combinations actually have caused problems, so it's probably best to avoid any that can potentially be harmful. Be especially cautious if you are on any type of blood-thinning or anticoagulant medication. Talk to your doctor about herbs you would like to try, find a pharmacist who's up on herbal remedies, and ask whether the ones you take can interact with your prescription medications.

Homeopathy

Homeopathy is a system of health care and treatment that was developed in 1796 by Dr. Samuel Hahnemann in Germany. The philosophy of homeopathy is based on Hahnemann's research with natural medicines in which he found that "like cures like." A substance causing certain symptoms in a healthy person can cure a sick person with the same symptoms. This theory is based on the belief that the body enlists its own energies to heal itself and defend against illness. If a substance that causes symptoms similar to those of the illness is administered, the body steps up its fight against it, thereby promoting cure.

> ## A Reminder
> Do not discontinue any prescribed medications without consulting your physician. And be sure always to tell your medical physician about any complementary or alternative therapies you decide to use.

The substances may be made from plants such as aconite or dandelion; from minerals such as iron phosphate, arsenic oxide, or sodium chloride; from animals such as venom of a number of poisonous snakes or the ink of the cuttlefish; or even from chemical drugs such as penicillin or streptomycin. These substances are diluted carefully until little of the original remains.

The National Center for Homeopathy (NCH) tells us that although most homeopathic medicines are available without a prescription, they are drug products made by homeopathic pharmacies, and their manufacture and sale are closely regulated by the Food and Drug Administration (FDA). Each individual state regulates the practice of homeopathy. Usually it can be employed legally by those whose degree entitles them to practice medicine in that state. This includes the M.D. (medical doctor), D.O. (doctor of osteopathy), N.D. (doctor of naturopathy), D.D.S. (dentist), and D.V.M. (veterinarian). Homeopathic practitioners can also include chiropractors, nurse practitioners, physician assistants, acupuncturists, and certified nurse midwives.[13] To find a licensed practitioner near you, search the NCH Membership Directory and Homeopathic Resource Guide, or visit its Web site at www .homeopathic.org.

Jennifer Gaddy, N.D., believes that together with a variety of therapies that heal by addressing the mind and body, homeopathy can be very helpful to people with fibromyalgia. "There are over-the-counter homeopathic remedies," she says, "that you can buy in most health food stores. These homeopathic preparations can be of two main types: single-remedy preparations or combination homeopathic medications which contain anywhere from five to ten very common remedies for the symptom in the hope that one of these medications is the right one for the individual who takes it." Dr. Gaddy feels that sometimes these over-the-counter remedies work out fine, but she believes that, especially in the case of fibromyalgia, it's much more appropriate to have a trained homeopathic practitioner review the case in detail and prescribe medicines appropriate to your situation; this approach is called *constitutional homeopathy*.

Although most homeopathic medicines are available without a prescription, they are drug products made by homeopathic pharmacies and their manufacture and sale are closely regulated by the Food and Drug Administration.

"A *constitutional remedy* is a homeopathic medicine that is prescribed based on the homeopathic view of the most clearly individual qualities of the patient's experience of the illness," says Dr. Gaddy. "In the language of homeopathy, these qualities are called the SRP or 'strange, rare, peculiar' aspects of that person's experience of the illness."

Dr. Gaddy summarizes the process of homeopathic treatment by describing the prescription process: "A classical homeopath prescribes a constitutional homeopathic remedy only after a long interview with the patient that gives the practitioner a clear understanding of the symptoms. The practitioner also receives a detailed, holistic sense of the individual by asking questions spanning the patient's physical, mental, emotional, and spiritual experiences of life; this portrait of the patient is used to scrupulously differentiate between medicines." Dr. Gaddy heartily recommends this individualized approach to homeopathy.

If you'd like to first try over-the-counter homeopathic remedies (with the understanding that they may not be as effective as those that would be prescribed by a trained practitioner), Dr. Gaddy recommends you test the waters with the following types that are all sublingual (pellets placed under the tongue) and should be taken without food and drink and only as needed. Most over-the-counter homeopathic remedies come in the dosage strength called 30C. This is a fairly high strength, so you should sense a shift in symptoms after about three doses; if not, then you should stop taking it.

Kali carbonicum (Kali carb)

If you fall asleep easily but wake up between 3:00 and 5:00 A.M., you might try this remedy if the following description fits you. You may be a person who generally experiences anxiety during the day or upon waking, felt either in the stomach or as palpitations in the chest. You like things in order and are highly responsible. Duty is important to you, and you prefer to see things in black-and-white terms. You may feel fear and chilliness and may experience digestive and respiratory problems. You crave salt, sweets, and fats. You can tend to linger in situations that cause emotional angst and complain about them. You may have difficulty fully expressing feelings due to a sense of responsibility or desire to stay in control.

Kali phosphoricum (Kali phos)

Similar to *Kali carb*, if this medicine is right for you, you may be a person who wakes between 3:00 and 5:00 A.M. You have a lingering sense of disorientation and mental fogginess, with sensitivity to your environment; you may feel jumpy or be easily startled. You may often feel chilled but crave cold drinks, particularly cold milk. *Kali phos* is used often in cases of nervous exhaustion, in which the individual has gone through a period of intense stimulation or tension and has become drained by this experience. There is usually a left-sidedness (worse on the left side) aspect to physical symptoms.

Calms forte

This combination homeopathic remedy is best if you can't fall asleep to begin with. The remedies used in this preparation are very mild and yet for some very effective. Take this medicine when you're having trouble getting to sleep. Take one dose as you go to bed. Take another a half hour later if you are still awake. And take another an hour later if needed. After three to five doses, you should know whether this therapy is going to help you.

Lycopodium

If your fatigue is at its worst in the late afternoon (between 4:00 and 8:00 P.M.), you are a person who craves sweets, and you have a sense of deep insecurity (although to others you appear self-secure), you could benefit from *lycopodium*. You may have a fear of failure and have some degree of digestive disturbance, with a tendency for gas. A strong intellectual tendency with a desire to prove to others is often seen in this remedy. It is dubbed by some as "the teacher's remedy."

Sulfur

A sulfur constitutional type often is highly responsible and possesses a sometimes rapid pacing in work. Usually the person has a firm sense of confidence on the level of business and work. There can be an experimental quality or free-mindedness expressed in some aspect of work or personal life. There is a strong tie to family and even a difficulty moving on from these ties when it is perhaps appropriate.

Sulfur is a warm-blooded type, with a large thirst as well as appetite. Cravings are for spicy foods (sometimes with eccentric food-combining tendencies), as well as sweet and fatty foods, and thirst may be for cold drinks. Sulfur may go for long intervals without feeling thirsty and then suddenly be seized by thirst and drink in long gulps. Physically such a person can have a ruddy, rosy complexion. A keynote symptom for sulfur is sleeping with the feet or a leg out of the covers, even during the cold season; this type likes the cold side of the pillow and loves cool, fresh air.

> **Learn More**
>
> For more detailed information, Dr. Gaddy recommends the book *Homeopathic Self-Care: The Quick and Easy Guide for the Whole Family* by Robert Ullman, N.D., and Judyth Reichenberg-Ullman, N.D., M.S.W. (Prima, 1997).

Ignatia

This remedy may help your muscle pain if the pain feels better with the application of pressure—if you feel the strong need to press on your head when you have a headache and this actually eases the pain. *Ignatia* is helpful when there is a strong tendency to suppress emotion, even with a desire to have an emotional release but an inability to access the feeling. This type often experiences a lump-in-the-throat sensation, with an "uptight" feeling in the body, and suffers from spasms in muscles.

> Ignatia *may help your muscle pain if the pain feels better with the application of pressure.*

One needing *Ignatia* may experience moods, with periods of brooding closely cycling with gaiety. In terms of the onset of this person's illness, there is a strong relationship with having experienced a deep grief or trauma. It is viewed as a remedy for the emotionally confusing effects of deep disappointments.

Lachesis

This remedy should be tried if you are extremely sensitive to touch with any feeling of physical constriction being very uncomfortable; snug waistlines, turtlenecks, and even necklaces often are intolerable. The people who benefit most from this medicine are usually very talkative, and their talk has an emotional, even pressured, quality. They may also be inordinately suspicious people, often possessing sharp, clever, and sarcastic tongues. Their pain is worse on the left side.

Arnica

This remedy can be helpful for pain that feels bruised and sore. It's for those who say they feel like they've been hit. Its most common usage is for the prevention of bruising and inflammation following an acute physical trauma, although muscle pain that is similar in sensation to having been severely bumped or bruised often responds to this remedy as well. Try this remedy in lower strengths—for example, 6X, 12X, or 30X rather than 30C.

Searching for an Alternative Therapy

After exhausting conventional medical therapies like low-dose anti-depressants, 53-year-old Barbara turned to alternative therapies. "I went to a chiropractor for treatment for my headaches, but it didn't work for me. Massage was relaxing, but it did nothing to alleviate the most serious of my symptoms. Melatonin left a groggy after-effect. And although I've had great success using acupuncture for other things, it really didn't help my fibromyalgia. I was still getting two or three migraines a day, and the fatigue was still so bad I had trouble getting myself to the bathroom."

Then a homeopathist gave Barbara limomine. "I used 2 drops in a cup of distilled water three times a day, and, believe it or not, it was

Phosphoric Acid

Try phosphoric acid if you are not able to focus and feel brain fatigue. This remedy is indicated in an intuitive person who can take in too much from the environment and end up feeling completely washed out.

Massage

In his online article "Massage Therapy for Health and Fitness," Elliot Greene, M.C.T.M.B., who served as the national president of the American Massage Therapy Association from 1990 to 1994, says that the last 10 years or so have seen a proliferation of different terms, titles, and systems of massage: therapeutic, holistic, Swedish, sports, neuromuscular, bodywork, Oriental, shiatsu, acupressure, esalen, Reichian, polarity, and reflexology.[14] If you explore massage as an alternative therapy, remember that these are all different types of the same therapy.

Whatever the name, massage is much more than a relaxing luxury. Greene points out that the therapeutic benefits of massage are numerous:

unbelievably helpful. The bloating, fatigue, headaches, allergies, and digestive problems all eased. I also found great relief from my fibromyalgia symptoms when my gynecologist gave me a prescription for estrogen-progesterone hormones for menopause-related problems. My fatigue, my headaches, my allergies—all of my symptoms have benefited from these hormones. I've now gone back to work as a secretary, and I feel much better about 3 weeks out of every month, but the week before my menstrual period, I start to drag." Like many women who have noticed a connection between the severity of their symptoms and their menstrual cycle, Barbara wonders whether her flares are related to changing hormone levels.

- **Massage causes changes in the blood.** The oxygen capacity of the blood can increase 10 to 15 percent after massage.

- **Massage affects muscles throughout the body.** It can loosen contracted, shortened muscles and can stimulate weak, flaccid muscles. This muscle "balancing" can help posture and promote more efficient movement. Massage also provides a gentle stretching action to both the muscles and connective tissues that surround and support muscles and many other parts of the body, which helps keep these tissues elastic.

- **Massage can increase the body's secretions and excretions.** There is a proven rise in the production of gastric juices, saliva, and urine. There is also increased excretion of nitrogen, inorganic phosphorus, and sodium chloride (salt). This suggests that the metabolic rate (the utilization of absorbed material by the body's cells) increases.

- **Massage can affect the nervous system.** It balances the nervous system by soothing or stimulating it, depending on which effect is needed by the individual at the time of the massage.

- **Massage can affect internal organs.** By indirectly or directly stimulating nerves that supply internal organs, blood vessels of these organs dilate and allow greater blood supply to them.

- **Massage can counter the effects of stress.** Stress can reduce circulation and interfere with digestion.[15]

In addition to these general benefits, Clifford Korn, N.C.T.M.B., who is a massage therapist at Windham Health Center Neuromuscular Therapy in New Hampshire, believes that massage is one of the therapies more commonly used by people with fibromyalgia that actually makes a difference in the way they feel. "What happens physiologically to make that so, I can't say," he admits. "But I do know that in my experience, people with fibromyalgia who use massage therapy do often say that it is one of the few things that makes them feel better—even though it may be only for a day, or in some cases, a matter of several days. It does have a positive effect."

> *Massage is one of the therapies more commonly used by people with fibromyalgia that actually makes a difference in the way they feel.*

Korn says that he remembers one client in particular, named Joan, who had remarkable results. "I met this woman when a colleague and I set up a massage chair in a local pharmacy to promote our business. She said that she had fibromyalgia and had been thinking about trying massage, and even though she was visiting New Hampshire only for the summer, she would like to come in for a consultation. At our first meeting, I learned that Joan had loved to square dance but found a while ago that after about 20 minutes she would have to stop because her joints would ache so much. And now she couldn't do it at all. Her goal was to find a way to ease her pain so she could go back to square dancing."

Korn admits that he didn't have any grandiose ideas that he would be able to help her do that, but he was willing to give it a try. Joan came in weekly and soon brought with her stories of her new square-dancing adventures. She was back on the floor and loving it. Joan became a weekly regular throughout that summer. Then Korn recalls, "At the end of the summer, I noticed that while I was doing her massage, she was crying. I put my hand on her shoulder and asked if everything was all right. She told me that the massage therapy was the first thing in 4 years that had an impact on her quality of life, and it probably kept her from committing suicide. This was when I first realized how much people suffering from fibromyalgia need understanding care."

But Korn acknowledges that caring for people with fibromyalgia requires a cautious approach and continual feedback from his clients. "If someone comes in and tells me he or she has this illness, I will spend time evaluating the specific symptoms, which can be as different as each one who walks through the door. Some will require a very superficial, light touch massage; they can't take a lot of pressure on the skin or joints. Others like very deep tissue work and they don't feel any benefit without it. It's important to find out how their discomfort manifests itself in the body and then decide what kind of massage would be best. Often we can't tell if a certain kind of massage will cause more discomfort or will ease the pain until we try it. Someone might tell me to do deep muscle work, but then tell me that discomfort from the massage lasted for 2 days. That lets me know I need to try something different. I need the client to tell me how the massage feels while I'm doing it and also to tell me how it feels the next day or two."

> Caring for people with fibromyalgia requires a cautious approach and continual feedback.

Korn notes that massage can be uncomfortable but should never be painful. "If someone is looking to effect a physical change in the body," he says, "the comfort is going to be based on the condition of the neuromuscular system in that body. If you have a muscle that is tight and I add pressure to it, that's going to have a certain degree of discomfort to it. But *discomfort* isn't a weasel word for pain. Massage should not be painful, and you need to tell your therapist if you feel pain."

Like many other therapies, how often and for how long you will need massage depends on your individual condition. Korn suggests several sessions per week, or at least no less than three visits in the first 2 weeks. "This gives the therapist fresh feedback," he explains, "and if there is a change, you're not going to revert back to ground zero by the time you come in for another session. This schedule also lets the therapist build on any progress. Then, 48 hours after the third session, you should do a little self-assessment. Ask yourself how you feel—any different? Any worse? Any better? That will help you and the massage therapist decide what kind of schedule makes sense for you.

> *Like many other therapies, how often and for how long you will need massage depends on your individual condition.*

"The goal is to make progress and begin spreading out the session to about once a week and then once every other week, and then reassess again," Korn explains. "When you get to a monthly massage and feel pretty good in between, you're on a maintenance schedule and can decide whether you want to continue or not."

The benefit you receive from massage therapy depends on the skill and training of the therapist. Do not use the yellow pages to find this person. Inconsistencies in national accreditation and licensing make it difficult to obtain a guarantee that everyone listed in the phone book is really a trained therapist. It's also risky because, unfortunately, some shady escort services advertise under the heading of "massage." The best method of finding a good therapist is through a medical or word-of-mouth referral.

Nutrition

A diet built on nutritious foods is vital in any treatment program for fibromyalgia. What you put into your body to feed and nourish all the cells, tissues, muscles, bones, and body systems has a direct effect on the severity of your symptoms. Brian Clement, the internationally renowned director of Florida's Hippocrates Health Institute and author of the book *Living Foods for Optimum Health*, has seen firsthand how diet can ease the pain and fatigue of this condition.

To use diet as a first-line therapy in the treatment of fibromyalgia, Clement recommends a vegetarian "living-foods" diet. He explains that like all vegetarian diets, a living-foods diet improves health and well-being by eliminating meat and dairy products. This first step automatically cleans the veins and arteries of fat and reduces the buildup of protein deposits. But unlike other vegetarians, living-food vegetarians thrive on the health-promoting components of oxygen, bioelectricity, enzymes, and alkalinity not found in cooked and processed foods.

Clement believes that living foods have the advantage over cooked foods as therapeutic substances for several reasons:

> **Referral Resource**
>
> For names of qualified massage therapists in your area, contact:
>
> **American Massage Therapy Association**
> 820 Davis Street, Suite 100
> Evanston, IL 60201
> Phone: (847) 864-0123
> E-mail: info@inet.amta massage.org
> Web site: www.amta massage.org

- Living foods increase the electromagnetic frequency of the cell. This replenishes the necessary bioactive alkaline and acid elements to keep cellular energy high and acid waste products low. The result is a strong immune system that can rejuvenate life within the cells of the body.

- Living foods provide the nutrients necessary to substantially develop a healthy tissue mass in all the body's organs, and they contribute to a healthier neurological sheathing and system so necessary to withstand the onslaught of fibromyalgia.

- Living foods reduce lethargy and increase energy because they contain high amounts of easy-to-digest amino acids.

The Power of Touch

"I was diagnosed with fibromyalgia in February 1991," says Bill of Plano, Texas. "I took a traditional route: multiple doctors, lots of physical therapy, lots of pain medication, light exercise, and mild stretching. I felt awful physically for the first 5 years, until I found the power of touch via massage. Regular massage has restored my ability to enjoy life. I receive massages twice a month on average, and I've made it a line item on my annual budget. It's part of every vacation I take. My massage therapist knows my body so well I can just stand in a room, and he'll say, 'So, you hurt right . . . here.' And he nails it every time. In my case, I've found that my muscular pain can be overcome through persistent stretching, lightweight resistance, improved nutrition, and, most important, massage."

- Living foods replenish the body's enzyme account. Food enzymes are depleted during the cooking process, which leaves the body prone to diseases and chronic illness.

- Living foods supply life-giving oxygen to the body's cells. Processed foods contain no oxygen, and even oxygen-rich foods lose their oxygen content when cooked. Deprived of an adequate supply of oxygen, the body becomes ripe for disease.

- Living foods also help the body detoxify to clean out the channels of elimination. This detoxification opens up the circulatory system, improves organ functions, and increases the water content of the body—all of which reduce potential stimulus for pain and increase normal function of all body systems.

There is no doubt that a diet that emphasizes living foods can revitalize, reenergize, and strengthen the body and its systems, and, according to Clement, it can also be a very effective therapy for the treatment and sometimes even the cure of fibromyalgia. "We've seen people who visit the Hippocrates Health Institute and follow our program of living foods who completely recover from fibromyalgia," says Clement, "but it can take a long time to rebalance the body, so you have to be vigilant and patient."

> *It can take a long time to rebalance the body, so you have to be vigilant and patient.*
>
> —BRIAN CLEMENT

You can begin a living-foods diet by eliminating animal products and slowly adding more fresh, uncooked vegetables, nuts, grains, and fruits to your daily diet. You should strive to eat about 70 percent of your foods in their natural state.

If you're not ready, willing, or able to make the switch to a living-foods diet, you can still help your body deal with the onslaught of the harmful substances you eat each day that aggravate the symptoms of fibromyalgia. Clement recommends the following:

- Switch to an organic-based diet. The pesticides, fungicides, and herbicides, along with the toxic effects of estrogens and biogenetically engineered foods, wreak havoc on the body.

- Reduce if not eliminate the amount of animal fat you take in.

- Increase the amount of healthful liquids you take in each day: switch to purified water, fresh juices, decaffeinated drinks, and herbal teas.

- Eliminate alcohol to ease the stress on the neurological system, which is already involved in perpetuating the symptoms of fibromyalgia.

- Eliminate caffeine and nicotine; they gunk up the system with waste products and interfere with healthy functioning of all body systems.

- Reduce if not eliminate processed foods; they are filled with things like white sugar, preservatives, and many other toxic chemicals that your sensitized body cannot handle without pain and disease.

- Be aware that part of your daily "diet" is also what you inhale in your environment. Buy nontoxic paints (now readily available in many name-brand varieties). Use woolen or cotton area rugs rather than wall-to-wall polyester formaldehyde carpeting. Do not buy clothes that need to be dry-cleaned. Make sure air circulates in your environment: Always keep a window cracked in the office and at home. Open your car window just a bit even when it's cold to counter the carbon monoxide continually coming into the car.

> *Your goal in using diet as a treatment therapy for fibromyalgia is to feed your body only foods that will nourish and support optimum health.*

Your goal in using diet as a treatment therapy for fibromyalgia is to feed your body only foods that will nourish and support optimum health. Give your body what it craves to be strong and healthy, and eliminate the foods and substances that overburden it with waste and debris.

BEWARE QUACKERY

Access to instant, global information through our computers brings us innumerable remedies and therapies for the treatment of fibromyalgia. In seconds, we can access medical research files from major universities. We can explore the Web sites of national and international organizations and find directories and referral programs. We can talk through online chat rooms to others who have fibromyalgia and discuss what works and what doesn't in treating this complex illness. This abundance of information has opened many doors to people with fibromyalgia who just a few years ago had such little information. But it has also opened the door to the fraudulent scams and hoaxes of those who prey on desperate people with chronic conditions.

Dr. John Astin, who received his Ph.D. in health psychology from the University of California, Irvine, before taking his current position as a researcher for the Complementary Medicine Program at the University of Maryland School of Medicine, feels that people with chronic, incurable conditions have good reason to seek alternative measures—but with caution. He believes you have to take the time to research what you're getting into. "Getting information is easier than ever before with the Internet," says Dr. Astin, "but you should stick to reputable sites. You can use a site like www.medline.com, for example, to search for information on any medication, procedure, therapy, or remedy and find out in seconds what has been studied on this subject. Then you can use your own best judgment to decide what's best for you."

While doing this research, Dr. Astin says that if he were a patient looking for an alternative therapy, he'd keep these guidelines in mind:

- Be highly critical of a product that offers a cure for fibro-myalgia—at this point in time there is no known, studied, or verified cure.

- Be skeptical of a product that offers relief of the symptoms without any legitimate research behind the claim.

- Beware of research that is based on a clinical trial sponsored by the manufacturer's own company rather than an independent facility like a university.

- Begin with therapies for which there is some documented, scientific evidence of effectiveness.

With these "buyer beware" warnings understood, Dr. Astin is quick to agree that many remedies that have not yet been studied or clinically proven might be very effective in treating the symptoms of fibromyalgia. "Given the plethora of options out there and the fact that we haven't researched 99.9 percent of them," says Dr. Astin, "consumers are faced with a dilemma. If I had fibromyalgia, I'd have to be open-minded about experimenting with different therapies—provided I'm not spending my life savings, and I feel some assurity about the safety of a product. If you are suffering and conventional medical practice hasn't been able to offer you relief, the best way to find what's right for you is to use your body as your personal laboratory. If the risk is low, why not experiment?"

Whatever you decide to try, it is a good idea to let your physician know about it. "There is increasing evidence," says Dr. Astin, "that things like 'natural' supplements and herbs and neutraceuticals are not benign substances; they have active compounds in them that can interact with other medications. So your doctor needs to know what you're taking. If your doctor is not open to experimentation and you want to experiment, then you do not have the right physician."

If you do your research first, assure yourself of a product's safety, and talk to your medical doctor about it, you should be able to avoid alternative therapies that are really nothing more than quackery and save your time and money for those that offer some realistic promise of relief.

WHEN IT WORKS, IT REALLY WORKS

Thirty-year-old Maria is a journalist who has fibromyalgia. She says she feels like she has been on a Sherlock Holmes detective trail trying to find out what's going on inside her body and how she can make herself feel better.

"I know all kinds of things can trigger a fibromyalgia flare-up," says Maria. "In my case, I think there are a number of factors I have to deal with. When I mentioned to my pain specialist—a chiropractor and kinesiologist—that I had been exposed to mercury on a daily basis while working for my father in the summers during high school and college, he decided I should have a hair analysis done. (I worked for my dad, who was a dentist, at a time when we mixed mercury and silver together for amalgam fillings and squeezed the excess mercury through a cloth.) The hair analysis revealed that I have a higher than normal mercury level in my system, and so my pain specialist will be treating me with something to help eliminate the mercury.

"In addition to the hair analysis," Maria continues, "he also suggested a fecal analysis, which showed that I had an overgrowth of yeast in my intestinal tract. I wasn't surprised to hear this because I had a problem with recurring vaginal yeast infections with no outward cause, and the infections were unresponsive to conventional treatment. My pain specialist recommended *Uva ursi*, a natural plant extract, as well as *Lactobacillus acidophilus*, which I took for about a month. With that treatment, I have rebalanced the flora and fauna in my intestinal tract, and that seems to have helped a lot."

Maria also had her blood tested for food allergies. "What I found was amazing," she says. "It turns out I react badly to sugar and the nightshade vegetables (tomatoes, potatoes, green peppers, eggplant, cabbage). I eliminated them from my diet for 6 months, and this made a big difference. Although I am less successful eliminating sugar because I crave it, I do notice that if I stay away from the nightshade vegetables, I feel much better. I've started to slowly reintroduce the vegetables, but I find that when I try them, especially tomatoes, the pain returns. For me there is definitely a relationship between these foods and my pain from fibromyalgia."

Initially, Maria went to a support group for fibromyalgia but found it depressing. "So many of the people there were on heavy-duty pain relievers, and they defined themselves as disabled," she remembers. "I think attitude makes a big difference in the way this disease feels, and all I heard was, 'Oh, poor me; I'm going down the tubes.' Then I thought, 'I'm not going to be defined by this condition. I'm not going to let it ruin my life, and I'm not going to get on pain medication.' That's when I went on my quest to find alternative ways to deal with this."

> *Okay, this is a challenge for me to meet, but I'm going to have a fabulous life regardless.*
>
> —MARIA

After trying a number of therapies, Maria has settled on regular exercise, meditation, massage, chiropractic adjustments, and supplements. "Because I'm a writer and editor, I sit in front of a computer all day—which is the worst thing I can do for this condition," Maria admits. "Most of my tension and pain is in my neck and shoulders, and I often find my shoulders hiked up around my ears. So I use an exercise system called Pilates to retrain my body while I stretch and strengthen muscle groups. Pilates shifts the tension from my neck and shoulders by helping me find my center in my abdominal muscles and strengthening them. In general, I find that the more exercise I get, the better I feel. The more I work out, the less pain I have.

"My pain specialist is an expert in body biochemistry and uses both chiropractic adjustments and kinesiology to help me when my fibromyalgia flares up. Through kinesiology, he can determine which supplements might help by testing certain supplements on my tongue.

"He has me lie on a table," Maria explains, "and he places a substance—usually in powder form—like vitamin C, on my tongue, which immediately triggers the nerve pathways to the muscles he's testing. Then he tests my muscle reaction. He might, for example, ask me to hold up my arm or leg while he tries to push it down. When I first experienced this technique, it amazed me that when he put one substance on my tongue, I could push back against his pressure, but with another substance, my muscles might feel weak, and I wouldn't be able to hold my arm or leg steady."

Based on this kind of testing, Maria takes several supplements to support her health. "I now take homocysteine metabolite, which gets rid of the buildup of homocysteine in the body. I also take 1,000 milligrams of vitamin C twice a day, a B-complex vitamin, and vitamin E with selenium and magnesium malate."

Maria also takes Coenzyme Q_{10}, which is another antioxidant. "Anecdotally, I heard that a lot people with fibromyalgia use CoQ_{10}," Maria says. "Because it's not harmful, I thought I might as well try it.

I can't say for sure if it's made a difference or not, but it seems like a good idea in general to take an antioxidant, so I've stuck with it."

Although she still has periods when she re-lapses into generalized pain, the times when Maria feels good and normal are lengthening. "If I manage my stress and my diet, and if I get exer-cise and take my supplements, I really feel very good. Actually, in a way having fibromyalgia has been a gift to me. I've lost 15 pounds by watch-ing my diet and exercising, so I'm back to the size I was in college. And I'm generally much

> *A lthough she still has periods when she relapses into generalized pain, the times when Maria feels good and normal are lengthening.*

healthier overall; I'm rarely sick. FMS has forced me to make lifestyle changes that are good for anyone, with or without fibromyalgia, and I'm really much better for it."

Maria is right. Finding the right therapies for fibromyalgia can be like playing Sherlock Holmes. But for those like Maria who have put in the time and effort, the benefits are astounding. As you search for the CAM therapies that will improve the quality of your life, remem-ber this one guideline: No one treatment is going to be a magic cure. The treatment of fibromyalgia requires an integration of your physi-cal, mental, emotional, and spiritual life.

Dealing with fibromyalgia can also require that you adjust the way you interact with your spouse, friends, and colleagues. Chapter 7 will explore this side of chronic illness.

CHAPTER 7

Fibromyalgia and Life Relationships

Arming yourself with information about the symptoms, diagnosis, and treatment of fibromyalgia is a vital part of finding a way to deal with this chronic disorder. But after all the facts are in, life goes on and you'll find that the next hurdle to jump is the one built on the many relationships you've established in your life. You'll quickly find that you do not have fibromyalgia in a vacuum. Everyone around you is affected by your health. Your spouse, significant other, children, friends, coworkers, and employers all have to live with the reality that your chronic health condition affects the way you function, the way you feel physically and emotionally from one day to the next, and the way you relate to each one of them.

FAMILY LIFE

It is a sad fact that chronic conditions like fibromyalgia can tear a family apart. This is especially true if the relationships were formed during a time of good health. If you married or built a life with a significant other before FMS, you established a relationship based on the assumption that you would be a happy, healthy life partner, but now that has changed. Your illness requires everyone to rethink daily responsibilities, and sometimes this leads to resentment and anger. Maybe you used to do most of the daily chores and child-care tasks, and now you need more help. Maybe you used to do the grocery shopping and wash the dishes, and now the shelves are often bare and the dishes piled up in the sink. The anger, resentment, and guilt that these kinds of changes can cause can throw a relationship into a tailspin that can be hard to recover from.

> *Your illness requires everyone to rethink daily responsibilities, and sometimes this leads to resentment and anger.*

Cameron Preece, Ph.D., a marriage and family therapist in group practice with Psychological Health Care, PLLC, is also a researcher from Syracuse University, New York, who has been studying the effects of family relationships on fibromyalgia for a study entitled "The Relationship Between Family Resilience and the Successful Management of Fibromyalgia." He has found that the success rate of the treatment plans commonly prescribed for fibromyalgia (e.g., medication, physical therapy, and cognitive restructuring) are significantly affected by the degree of support the person with FMS receives from his or her spouse or significant other. Family understanding seems to magnify the effects of many treatment modalities; it is related to the severity of the symptoms, the amount of medication a person uses, and whether a person can effectively use pain-coping mechanisms.

Dr. Preece explains:

> In a typical scenario, a woman with fibromyalgia comes in, and we set up a treatment program for her. Then we find that every time she has a flare, her husband berates her and tells her it's all in her head. When that happens, the effects of all the exercise, and coping techniques, and relaxation therapies is diminished because what she really needs to feel well is to feel that her husband loves her and accepts her for who she is.

To make treatment therapies work successfully for the patient, I have learned to work with the patient's husband as well, to help him understand and accept his wife's illness. Focusing solely on the medical needs of someone with fibromyalgia is only a part of the picture. This psychosocial research for this condition is really cutting-edge and very exciting. Of course, it's only a start and there's a lot more to learn, but these initial findings are very important.

> *There's no doubt that the way your family lives with your fibromyalgia will have a strong effect on how you live with it, too.*

Dr. Preece's work fills in another piece of the fibromyalgia puzzle. You cannot ignore what's going on in your family and focus only on your symptoms and medical treatments. There's no doubt that the way your family lives with your fibromyalgia will have a strong effect on how you live with it, too.

Getting Past the Trials and Tribulations

Paula had been married 8 years when she was diagnosed with fibromyalgia at age 28. It took another 6 years before she and her husband and two sons learned how live with it.

"We had a lot of adjusting to do. When my husband and I married, he didn't sign on for this kind of relationship," admits Paula. "At first I was having trouble with depression, sleep problems, and some muscle spasms in my shoulder, but nothing that really interfered with my family life. But then the pain increased dramatically. My hips began to ache, and the pain in my spine was unbearable. I left my job as a cashier because I couldn't lift anything anymore. I went back to school and graduated first in my class as a hairdresser. But standing on my feet all day hurt my hips so bad that it was hard to walk. My doctor prescribed morphine, hoping that would help me to keep working. But I recently had to leave that job, too.

"My husband and I were both worried about how we would manage financially, but he never complained to me. He says I don't need anybody else to beat up on me—I do enough of that to myself. He's right. I hate not being able to work. I hate not being able to take my kids out ice skating. But I'm very lucky to have my husband's support. If I'm having a bad day, he takes over without saying a word. He has been fantastic, and things are very good for us now, but I have to admit that they weren't that way at first."

In the beginning, Paula's husband believed that if they didn't talk about her physical problems, they would go away. "That was very frustrating, and it was hard on the marriage," says Paula. "We never really talked about it, and it caused a lot of unspoken anger and resentment for both of us." Paula feels this very difficult time began during the 2 years she needed morphine to continue working. "It wasn't until I stopped taking the morphine and he saw how real the pain was that he was able to understand. When my pain was masked by the painkiller, I don't think he could imagine what I was going through. But once he saw it for himself, he knew I needed his help, and that has actually brought us a lot closer. Having his support means everything to me."

Forty-one-year-old Pat, who works in corporate communications for a pharmaceutical company, has traveled across this same family battlefield. "It has been very challenging to get to this point as a family," says Pat, "where my husband is now understanding and is a big help to me. He knows I need to do things because of my illness, like take time to relax, take a warm bath, do stress reduction exercises, and things like that. He's learned to understand my needs, and he knows that if he wants to have me continue to be available to him as a wife and a friend, then I need to be able to take care of myself first."

But, like Paula, it took Pat and her husband a long time to get to this point. "A year ago we lived a totally different life," remembers Pat. "It was a time of fear, frustration, and anger. My pain got so bad day in and day out that I was struggling to work full-time, keep up the house, and be the primary caregiver to our son. That's when we had a family huddle and decided that things had to change. I knew we all had reached the point where we couldn't take it anymore. Obviously this realization didn't happen overnight. There were a lot of trials and tribulations, arguments, fighting, resentment, and all the things that go with this kind of family change. It's not just the illness, but it's the need to reorganize your relationships so you can get on with your life that is very hard to do."

Pat found the way through this challenge with the help of professional physical and behavioral therapists. "At first I thought all our problems were my fault. I had to learn over time that it wasn't *me* that my family was resenting; it was my illness. I don't think I could have come to this realization on my own. I needed somebody on the outside to explain that to me and to reinforce it and help me accept it.

"It's very helpful to talk to someone who is trained to deal with people who have chronic illnesses," Pat notes. "Now I know I can live with this, but it has taken some life changes and some help to get on the right path."

Look at Both Sides of the Relationship

Getting on the right path is an important first step in finding a way to live with fibromyalgia. No one knows this better than Penney Cowan, executive director of the American Chronic Pain Association (ACPA) in Rocklin, California—who also has had fibromyalgia for 27 years. Penney has worked with many families who are living the reality of fibromyalgia and has seen how difficult it can be on everyone. In her book, *American Chronic Pain Association Family Manual*, Cowan says, "Consider the family where one person has been forced to reduce activity levels, working hours, and financial responsibility to almost nothing. Suddenly the burden of supporting the family financially, emotionally, and physically falls on the well spouse. What are the chances of this family surviving long term if they cannot communicate their needs and feelings?"[1]

We all know the odds are small. The person who can no longer do what he or she used to do feels frustrated, angry, and left out of the fun. The person who has to pick up the slack may feel let down, abused, and neglected. Children may feel afraid or even to blame.

Before writing this manual, Cowan interviewed families over a 3-year period. Her findings have helped her work with both the person in chronic pain and the family he or she lives with. "The family members are usually the forgotten ones," says Cowan. "I found that they suffer in very much the same way except for the physical symptoms. All the painful emotions, the lost plans and dreams, the anger and frustration are theirs, too." Cowan believes that very often people with chronic conditions like fibromyalgia don't realize that their loved ones are also struggling, and that's why they can't always be as supportive as they'd like to be.

> Very often people with chronic conditions like fibromyalgia don't realize that their loved ones are also struggling, and that's why they can't always be as supportive as they'd like to be.

Everyone in the family needs to learn how to acknowledge and communicate their emotional feelings. Everyone needs to be assertive and express personal feelings. When you're angry, or frustrated, or happy, you have to be able to say so. Everyone in the family needs to know what's going on with each other. Living with someone who has a chronic condition is difficult—there's no point in trying to hide that, yet so often family members hold all their feelings inside until they build up to the exploding point.

Once you realize that you are not the only one suffering from the effects of fibromyalgia, you can change the way you communicate with others. "Both sides need to acknowledge and validate that there are in fact real problems," says Cowan, "whether that's the pain and fatigue itself or the stress and confusion it causes. It's amazing how many walls can be quickly ripped down when people stop to acknowledge how another person is feeling and that both the person with fibromyalgia and his or her loved ones have problems to deal with." Cowan understands that it may be hard for you to feel empathy for your spouse who complains about having to do housework when you would love to do it if only your pain would stop screaming for attention, but she says it's important to listen to his or her feelings without feeling personally criticized.

A sample conversation of validation that you might try with your family members may sound something like this: "I feel very badly that I can't do all the things I used to do. And I understand that this change has been very hard on you, too. I want you to tell me about your feelings so we can work this out together." This kind of simple statement may open up doors of understanding and acceptance that have been long closed.

> *Once you realize that you are not the only one suffering from the effects of fibromyalgia, you can change the way you communicate with others.*

Avoid Talking About Physical Symptoms

It would be nice if caring family members could listen to your complaints of physical symptoms and come up with a way to "fix" you. But, unfortunately, that is not going to happen. Only the person with FMS can take the responsibility for living well. For this reason, Cowan encourages family members to avoid talking about physical symptoms. She feels it's best if family members don't start every conversation with, "How are you feeling?"

"This is a futile discussion because no one will ever really know how another person feels physically," explains Cowan. "We cannot measure our pain. We cannot take the pain out of the body and hold it in our hand and say, 'You really want to know how much I'm hurting? Here it is; this is how much I hurt.' Pain is invisible, so people in relationships with those who have chronic pain have to believe that the pain is real, but they shouldn't continually remind them and keep them in that disabled/patient type of role where they're not in control."

The person with fibromyalgia also needs to learn a new way of communicating that does not focus on fibromyalgia. You may have a natural inclination to want to make your loved ones understand how you feel. You want to say, "I feel awful; you just don't understand, and so I'm going to keep describing how I feel until you get it." "But," says Cowan, "no one will ever understand how you really feel, so it's a waste of time to keep telling everyone around you the details of the pain and fatigue that plague you. It is impossible to feel another person's pain, so don't get hung up trying to explain it. Even if you cut your finger and someone else cuts his finger in the same spot, you will still experience the pain in different ways."

> *People in relationships with those who have chronic pain have to believe that the pain is real, but they shouldn't continually remind them and keep them in that disabled/patient type of role.*
>
> —PENNEY COWAN

Talking about your pain is also counterproductive because if you have to keep explaining how you feel, you are forced to keep thinking about it. "The more you think about the pain," says Cowan, "the more you suffer. You're going to suffer less if you can redirect your thoughts off of the pain and onto something you have more control over. That doesn't mean your pain is going to miraculously go away; it means you won't suffer as much. The goal is to learn how to keep pain from becoming the focus of your life. This is the hardest hump to get over and accept."

Saying that you should avoid talking about your physical symptoms is not recommending that you enter a state of denial—just the opposite. Remember, you should start with a conversation that asks everyone in your family to acknowledge and validate your physical condition. Once you all agree that you are living in a very difficult circumstance, then there is no reason to keep going over and over that.

Develop a Family System of Communication

Once family members acknowledge and validate that you have physical symptoms that are difficult to deal with, you can then begin to change the way you all communicate. Cowan recommends that you establish a very neutral system that lets you communicate the way you feel at any given time without having to further justify, validate, or explain yourself. If your family wants to go ice skating and you know that a trip out in the cold will make your already aching muscles worse, you can simply say, "That's not something I can do today," without trying to make them understand all your reasons. Or, you can agree in advance that if you say, "This is a bad day," everyone will understand and accept your behavior without asking for an explanation.

> *Talking about your pain is also counter-productive because if you have to keep explaining how you feel, you are forced to keep thinking about it.*

There are many ways you can communicate without putting yourself in the patient role. Some members of the American Chronic Pain Association use communication systems that are based on our understanding of traffic lights, for example; this might be a green light day, or a red light day, or even a yellow light day of caution. Others draw little faces on the kitchen calendar with either a smile or a frown to let everyone know nonverbally where things stand that day. And everyone in the family has this same right. If your spouse has had a tough day and just can't get the kids bathed at night, he has to have the right to say so. If your significant other just doesn't feel like doing all the cooking again, she should be allowed to call for some take-out without having to justify or explain.

General Communication Tips

The skill of communicating feelings and needs may take some time to develop—especially if your present method is either to shout or to stop talking completely. The following communication tips, adapted from the *American Chronic Pain Association Family Manual*, will help you get started:

- **Avoid emotionally charged conversation.** Recognize how you feel emotionally before becoming involved in a serious discussion. When you or your listener are emotionally upset, it

Your Basic Rights

Penney Cowan, executive director of the American Chronic Pain Association, compiled this list of basic rights:

- You have the right to say no.

- You have the right to do less than what is humanly possible.

- You have the right not to have to justify your behavior.

- You have the right to be treated with dignity and respect.

may be difficult to concentrate or be objective. Sometimes timing is everything.

- **Make sure you are not in too much pain to concentrate or be objective.** When discussing an issue that is important to a family member, everyone needs to pay attention. Pain can decrease the ability to process what is being said. You may agree to what is being said at the time but, when your pain is under control, totally forget the conversation ever took place.

- **Take responsibility for what you say.** Whenever possible, try to speak in the first person. Avoid statements like, "We all know . . ." or, "So-and-so told me . . ." Your emotions and feelings are yours. Say, "I feel . . ." If you are sharing a thought, say, "I think that . . ." If you are making a request, say, "I want . . ." It is not appropriate to believe that someone else can infer what you feel, so it's important that you express your own ideas. And remember that your honest feelings are valid—you have a right to them.

- **Listen to the feedback others give you.** Three people in the room are all listening to the same discussion. If they were asked what they heard, it would not be unusual to hear three totally different ideas. When people listen, they listen with their ears, their experiences, and their emotions. To ensure that a message is understood, ask others their understanding of what was said. This gives you the opportunity to clarify any misinterpretations immediately and keep the lines of communication open.

- **Be direct about your needs.** There is a lot to be said for getting directly to the point. If you need something, simply ask.

- **Don't allow others to tell you how you feel.** Our feelings are unique. Unless we tell others how we feel, they have no way of knowing. If someone tells you how you feel, you have the right to state, in your own words, how you really feel. To ensure that people know how you feel, use statements that start with phrases such as, "I feel . . ." or "I think . . ."

- **You have no control over other people.** In spite of how well you communicate, in the end, you have no control over what others say, do, or think. Communication is only the beginning of action. To achieve the desired results, families must work together, respecting each other's point of view.

Talking to Children About Fibromyalgia

What you say to your children about fibromyalgia depends, of course, on their age. The important thing is that you do talk to them and keep on talking as they grow. Experts in child development know that you cannot "protect" your children with silence. You cannot make things easier for them by saying, "I'm just fine," when they ask, "What's the matter?" Like any other relationship in your life, if you want your relationship with

Communication Tools to Help You Express Yourself

- Use body language. Be relaxed in the way you move, stand, or sit. Positive body language reflects self-confidence.

- Personalize. Use "I" statements to take responsibility for what you are saying.

- Be direct and clear. Get right to the point and state exactly what you want.

- Recognize the circumstances of the individual of whom you are making a request.

- Be willing to compromise.

- Know that you will not always get everything you want.

Used with permission of Penney Cowan, American Chronic Pain Association Family Manual *(1998).*

your children to be strong, you have to give them enough information so they can understand why you may not always be able to run around and play like their friends' mommies or daddies.

If your child is old enough to understand the concept of being "sick," she is old enough to learn something about fibromyalgia. Dennis Turk, Ph.D., of the University of Washington in Seattle, suggests that you can tell your children about the two kinds of illnesses: some, like a cold or sore throat, that come once in a while but don't last long; and the kind that doesn't go away. Explain that there are chronic conditions like asthma, high blood pressure, diabetes, and so on, that many people have to learn to live with.

Dr. Turk advises:

You want to normalize the condition. You don't want your children to think you have something that's really weird and that may kill you.

Let them know that you are just like many people living with chronic conditions. Tell them that you have an illness called fibromyalgia that doesn't have a quick cure. You might say, "It's a condition that gets better for a while and then comes back again. There's not anything that I can do to get rid of it, but I am learning how to live better with it." The message is: "What I have is not different from many other chronic diseases, but it is different from the kind of illnesses that have a quick cure and then goes away. Although it can't be cured, there are things I can do to help me function better, but I will still have some limitations."

Explain that you are going to have some good days and some bad days. Promise your children that you'll tell them when you're having a bad day and what your limitations are on those days. You can also talk about the things they can do on your bad days that would help

> *Experts in child development know that you cannot "protect" your children with silence.*

you (like playing quietly) and the things that would make the day harder for you (like inviting all their friends over to make cookies). You have to talk about what's going on with information that's appropriate to their age level.

Your kids aren't mind readers who can know, or guess, or assume how you feel or how they can help you. So talk to them and keep the conversation going—this isn't a one-time conversation. Young kids won't remember what you told them a month ago, so be sure to remind them every once in a while how you feel, why you feel that way, and what both of you can do to make the situation better.

This is sound advice, but in reality some parents find it hard to talk to their kids about fibromyalgia. "I didn't want my boys, who are 13 and 15 years old, to worry about me," says Paula (who you'll remember from her story earlier in this chapter has had fibromyalgia for 8 years). "I never told them anything about my health, but I guess they noticed that something was wrong. When I first went off the morphine, I spent most of my days sitting in a chair (I couldn't even walk)—they couldn't have missed that. Now that I think about it, I guess they might even have worried that I had bone cancer like their grandma does."

Paula's eldest son now knows about his mother's illness, but only after a recent outburst. "I was sitting on the couch one night," remembers Paula, "and I asked my son to get something for me. He gave me an answer that was just not normal for him; he said, 'Why? Because you can't get off your lazy ass and get it for yourself?' When he later apologized for his words, Paula finally told him why she sometimes just can't get off the couch. "Since that time," says Paula, "he has been very understanding and very helpful to me. I think I should probably tell my younger son, too. Basically, my kids are in a one-parent family when they want to go out and do anything. I can't go out ice skating, or tobogganing, or partying. Their dad has to take them. I guess they should know why. What my younger son is imagining is wrong with me is probably worse than reality."

> *You want to normalize the condition. You don't want your children to think you have something that's really weird and that may kill you.*
>
> —DENNIS TURK, PH.D.

Paula's absolutely right. On their own, children will pick up very quickly that something is wrong, and, if left to their own imagination, they will usually imagine the worst. That's why Pat (the corporate communications manager introduced earlier) has made sure that her 7-year-old son has grown up knowing that his mommy has what he calls "fibro-algia." Pat was diagnosed with fibromyalgia when her son was 6 months old, so it has always been part of his family life.

"When Ryan was about 5 years old, it was a tough time for him," remembers Pat. "He would get really angry when I couldn't play with him. He'd say things like, 'You don't love me anymore. You're always sick. It's not fair!' That was especially difficult to work through until I realized I'd need to create a new kind of 'mommy time' that made us both happy.

"Instead of going to the park and doing physical things (I leave that up to his dad), I now spend more time with him doing less physical things. We snuggle in bed and read books together. I sit next to him and we watch cartoons. We spend time playing with his toys and playing board, video, and computer games. This is very good quality time for us. The times when I am just so tired or feeling like I can't even sit and watch TV, I explain to him that 'Mommy's muscles hurt.' He knows that I have an illness that makes my muscles hurt and sometimes I take medicine to feel better. He can now even judge my moods, and he knows when it's a good time to play and when it's not. There have even been times when he'll say, 'Mommy, I know you're not feeling good today, so let's just read books.' He's now at an age where he wants to help and console me, and he understands that I will feel better again soon.

> *On their own, children will pick up very quickly that something is wrong, and, if left to their own imagination, they will usually imagine the worst.*

"I just keep putting one foot in front of the other, and each day seems to get a little better for all of us."

FIBROMYALGIA AND YOUR SEXUALITY

Jane Greer, Ph.D., is a marriage, family, and sex therapist from New York City who writes the online column "Let's Talk About Sex" for Redbookmag.com. Dr. Greer has worked with several women who have had fibromyalgia, and she knows that because the web of FMS interacts with so many other aspects of life—from social, to work, to personal—that its effect on sexual intimacy often goes ignored and unspoken.

"The enormity of living with this illness causes its effect on sexuality to get lost in the mix," says Dr. Greer. "Its sexual effect deserves to be flushed out and recognized as substantive unto itself. A chronic condition like fibromyalgia can increase your threshold for pain and lower your threshold for pleasure, so soon you're having sex less often, and your partner becomes convinced that you no longer find

Guidelines for Talking to Kids

When you talk to your children about fibromyalgia, keep these guidelines in mind:

- Make sure your children know that fibromyalgia will not kill you.

- Explain that some days are not so bad and other days are really bad.

- Emphasize that this condition is not their fault.

- Be honest and admit that right now there is no cure.

- Be optimistic about your plans to live well and your hope that soon the medical community will find a way to make you feel much better.

- Encourage your children to ask questions and talk to you about their fears and worries.

- Admit that sometimes you may need your children to understand why you can't always do everything you'd like to do with them.

him [or her] desirable." This misunderstanding has pulled many relationships to pieces.

There is only one way to keep a sexual relationship strong when you have fibromyalgia: You have to talk about how the fatigue, pain, and complications of this condition affect your emotions, your feelings of sensuality, and your physical ability to have sexual intercourse. Remember, your partner cannot feel your pain; he cannot guess how certain positions put pressure on your tender points; he cannot know that your indifference to his advances has nothing to do with your feelings for him—he can't know unless you tell him. This is something that partners have to talk about.

Dr. Greer advocates open communication:

You need to communicate to your partner that you still have a desire to experience pleasure and that you need support to find new ways to tailor lovemaking so it can be enjoyable for both of you. You need to feel free to risk sexual activity knowing that if pain suddenly kicks in and disrupts your pleasure, your partner will understand that this doesn't mean you don't love him. He needs to know that you still find him attractive, even when you physically can't have sex.

Communicate that you care, that he still turns you on, that you're still interested in having sex with him, and that you're trying to find ways around the obstacles. These messages make a world of difference in the way your partner reacts to the adjustments he is being asked to make.

Here are a few tips that Dr. Greer suggests can help you maintain a strong relationship with your lover:

> *There is only one way to keep a sexual relationship strong when you have fibromyalgia: You have to talk about how the fatigue, pain, and complications of this condition affect your emotions, feelings of sensuality, and physical ability.*

- Tell your partner where your tender points are so he or she can avoid unintentionally causing you pain.

- Try a variety of positions—it's time to be creative and break old habits. Check out books and videos for advice on alternate positions that might make you feel more comfortable.

- Adjust your expectations. Don't define sex only as intercourse and orgasm.

- Focus more on sensual activities that feel good such as cuddling, soft massages, or a warm bath together.

- Be flexible in scheduling sexual encounters. If you don't feel up to it today, look forward to tomorrow.

- Help your partner feel sexually satisfied, even if you're not up to being sexually active yourself.

- Reassure your partner over and over that you still desire sex but sometimes get shut down by pain or fatigue.

- Talk. Talk about what feels good and what doesn't.
- Don't pressure yourself. Additional anxiety will not improve your sex life.

Dr. Greer believes that just as you must make accommodations in your schedule, on your job, and in your level of physical activity because you have fibromyalgia, you have to expect to make accommodations in your sexual life also. "It comes down to the fact that when you have fibromyalgia you have to alter your expectations, or you will constantly be disappointed that you can't always do what you used to do."

> **Side Effects and Sex**
>
> If your sex life is dragging, talk to your doctor about the side effects of your medications. Anti-depression and anti-anxiety medications can cause a decrease in sexual desire.

The Mental Part of Sexuality

A big part of sexuality is mental. How your partner feels about you and fibromyalgia can certainly affect how you feel about him or her in the bedroom. A supportive partner is a real turn-on, but a resentful, angry, or indifferent partner is like a cold shower. This is the dilemma that 27-year-old Rose is facing with her husband.

"I love my husband very much," says Rose, "but I get the feeling that he loves me only when I can smile and say, 'I'm just fine.' As soon as he sees that I'm in pain, he gets angry and storms out of the house. I don't dare say I'm too tired to do something, or he'll start yelling and calling me lazy. He just won't believe that there is something physically wrong with me. He can't get past the fact that all my tests come back negative. I'm finding it very hard to make love to someone who can't accept who I am."

Once again, talking openly and uncritically about your feelings—both yours and your partner's—is the first step in restoring emotional and therefore sexual balance between you. Validate each other's feelings, don't dwell on your own pain, and give yourselves time to readjust to what your body is forcing you both to accept.

WORK LIFE

Sometimes fibromyalgia has very little impact on a person's ability to work, but sometimes it forces a person out of a current job or out of work completely. When this happens, the financial and social impact can be devastating. That's why in most cases, the goal is to find a way to continue working without adding to the pain and discomfort of FMS.

To Tell or Not to Tell

Once you find out you have fibromyalgia, you may wonder, "Should I tell my coworkers and my boss?" Dr. Dennis Turk feels that the answer to that question depends on how your physical condition impacts on your ability to function:

> If it has relatively little impact, then tell very few people. If it were me, I wouldn't tell everyone I'm sitting around the coffee room with. But if a flare-up affects the way you do your job, then you need to tell people who work closely with you who may need to pick up the slack. If you have a supervisor who needs to know you need a rest period or an occasional break, then that person needs to know because no one is a mind reader. Unless your boss and close coworkers know you have fibromyalgia, they're likely to think you're lazy or slacking off or that you let other people do your work. Let them know what you have, how you're going to handle it, and how they can most effectively help you. Be direct and open with the people who need to know.

If you are able to continue performing your job responsibilities, you should not have to worry about being fired. Depending on your degree of symptom severity, the Americans with Disabilities Act (ADA) may help you retain or obtain employment if you think your job is in danger. The Civil Rights Division of the U.S. Department of Justice says that the ADA prohibits discrimination in all employment practices of individuals with physical or mental disabilities as long as the person meets legitimate skill, experience, education, or other requirements of an employment position and can perform the essential functions of the position. If your boss thinks FMS is cause for dismissal, be sure to contact the Department of Justice to verify your rights (see contact information below).

Making Life Easier at Work

It is worth the effort, time, and money to consult with an occupational therapist about your work environment—it can mean the difference between staying employed or quitting your job. This kind of therapist can tell you whether you need a more supportive chair or whether the desk height is causing muscle strain. Occupational therapists will find ways to keep you away from the air-conditioning duct or a drafty hallway. They can tell whether your body posture is aggravating your symptoms. They may suggest a phone rest, speakerphone, or headrest to ease the stress on your neck and elbow. Because you spend such a large part of your day in your work environment, it makes sense to be sure it is not working against you.

These kinds of changes have kept public relations/communications director Debby on the job longer than she originally thought possible. Although Debby didn't want to make her fibromyalgia a major work issue, she realized that to minimize her flares, she needed to make certain accommodations. "The company gave me a laptop computer that I really loved and needed, but it was just too heavy for me to carry around," says Debby. "I've learned that sometimes if I lift heavy objects, my symptoms can get really bad, even a day or two afterward. I especially worried about getting muscle pain from lugging the computer around when I was traveling. So the company gave me one that is much lighter.

Learn More

To obtain answers to general and technical questions about the Americans with Disabilities Act (ADA) and to order technical assistance materials, contact:

Department of Justice
Phone: (800) 514-0301
Web site: www.usdoj.gov
/crt/ada/adahom1.htm

"I also asked for a special kind of chair with back support. I was worried that they would think I was being a pain in the neck [no pun intended!], but they never gave me a problem. Lots of companies are becoming very good about supplying the necessary ergonomic office environments if you ask. For me, this is absolutely vital to my health and helps me do a better job for the company. This is one area where I think it's necessary to be very proactive."

It is worth the effort, time, and money to consult with an occupational therapist about your work environment—it can mean the difference between staying employed or quitting your job.

Changing Jobs

Many circumstances may make it impossible to work with fibromyalgia. To name just a few: A long commute can aggravate sore muscles. Standing long hours can be unbearable on painful feet, legs, and lower back muscles. The stress of a heavy travel schedule can cause continuous flares. Long hours can exacerbate the exhaustion that makes any kind of personal or social life impossible. Some jobs just are not compatible with fibromyalgia. But many people with FMS have found that there is a middle ground between working in misery and quitting. Here are a few changes people with FMS have successfully tried:

- **Ask for reassignment.** Sometimes there are jobs within the same company that are more compatible with FMS. Look into a lateral move.

- **Change jobs.** Find one that is closer to home, less stressful, or requires less travel.

- **Switch from full-time to part-time work.** If you can afford it, this options keeps you active and involved in life but gives you time to take care of yourself as well.

- **Telecommute.** Find a job that lets you join the millions of employees who now work from home.

- **Become an entrepreneur.** Starting your own business can let you work from home, set your own pace, and work around your good and bad days.

When the financial and social benefits you gain from employment are important to you, it's well worth the time and effort required to find a way to stay employed and yet acknowledge that to live well with fibromyalgia, you often have to make some adjustments.

Seeking a Slower Pace and Less Stress

Angie had a wonderful media job in news and promotion at an ABC-affiliate station in New Orleans. The job brought with it the excitement of writing, producing, shooting, editing, and squeezing under the wire to meet tight deadlines. It also brought late-night hours, lots of stress, and no time for self-care. Finally, in 1998, Angie's rheumatologist told her to rethink the value of this job—it was constantly feeding the pain of her fibromyalgia. "At that point, I was in so much agony I was willing to try anything."

Angie had been diagnosed with fibromyalgia in 1994. "When I first heard this crappy name for a condition I had never heard of, I went home and began to do my homework to find out as much as I could about it. I often read that stress made the symptoms worse, but I loved my job, and I just didn't want to let this problem change the way I lived my life. So I continued fighting the clock to put on quality news shows, and my pain and fatigue grew worse and worse."

At one point, Angie was getting injections of muscle relaxants and pain relievers once a week in her most painful tender points. But the difficulty of working and suffering from the symptoms of fibromyalgia became so bad that Angie took a 5-week leave of absence (at the urging of her boss, who told her outright, "You're looking bad"). At the start of those 5 weeks, Angie felt like she was going to die. She was sure something deadly was going on because she figured a chronic illness could not be so unbearable. She upped her injection

Getting the Job Done

When Debby interviewed for her job as a public relations/communications director, she decided that she would not mention that she had fibromyalgia—she would not let this condition define who she is and what she can do. But then shortly after being hired, just before she was to make her first presentation in front of her boss, Debby's muscles began to spasm. "I was in so much pain, but I still didn't tell anyone and went ahead with the presentation. Afterward, I wanted my boss to know that that wasn't my best. I remember saying, 'Just so you know, I was in tremendous pain in there. That's not how I would normally present. If you were happy with what I did, I'm glad—but that's not my best work.' I think that showed that I was not someone who would let fibromyalgia stop me from doing what I have to do. I can push through and get the job done. That's who I've decided I am."

schedule to twice a week, and then around the end of the third week, she turned a corner and felt a little better. She describes herself as a natural workaholic who can't just sit home waiting to feel better. After the 5 weeks were up, Angie headed back to work.

The pain and exhaustion level quickly became overwhelming once again. "Even though I was determined to push through this thing," Angie recalls, "I was walking around feeling like my ribs and collarbone were broken. I was also losing my train of thought, having trouble concentrating and feeling lots of fog in my head. I guess I was just being stubborn. I figured if this wasn't deadly, then I wasn't going to let it ruin my life. But when I look back now, I know I was pushing entirely too hard." Three years after her diagnosis, Angie left her job for another one that promised a slower pace and less stress.

Angie took a job as a broadcast producer at the University of Alabama in the office of media relations. Although the physical exertion required to pack up and relocate was tough on her physically, the effort was worth it. This job was very similar to her previous one, but the material she works with is generally all positive news, there are longer deadlines (she's no longer trying to put a show on the air three or four times a day), she works regular office hours, and this job allows her more time to be creative.

> *Although the physical exertion required to pack up and relocate was tough on Angie physically, the effort was worth it.*

Most important, this job change has changed the course of Angie's fibromyalgia. She now has more time to focus on her own well-being. "I now watch my diet and try to eat foods that support my health," she says. "I manage stress better now, too. When I'm in a stressful situation, I see what I can do and then know it's best to leave the rest behind. I've done more reading and talking about this condition and have learned where to set up my boundaries. I now have more time for a social life, too; before I spent my life in only three activities: working, sitting in the doctor's office, or sleeping. Now I have a real life."

Staying at home and feeling bad is not something Angie will even consider, but before she left her first job, her level of disability was so bad that she did not think she could live alone anymore. Still, she went to work every day. "Getting out and doing something constructive gave me a mental break from hurting and feeling like hell. Work is as nourishing to me as medication. If I sat at home, I personally would have fallen into a huge hole that would have put me into a very different kind of life than I have now."

Angie says she has had tremendous support from her family and friends and from her fibromyalgia support group as well. "The first group I joined was just horrible. It was nothing more than a whinefest. These people were not interested in holding onto life—they just wanted sympathy for their plight. But the second group I joined was good for me. It helped me evaluate resources that were available for me; it helped me sort through all the hype that's out there about fibromyalgia; it helped me avoid some scams and see a lot of the garbage that's out there. There's a lot of straight talk at these meetings, and they've helped me get through some tough times."

With her new job and a new support group, Angie is a new person. There is life after a diagnosis of fibromyalgia.

Work Disability

Among the many controversies surrounding fibromyalgia is the issue of work disability. Steve Thorson of the Fibromyalgia Network feels that disability for people with FMS is a very nebulous issue. "Disability is determined by, among other things, if you can show up consistently to work every single day and do all the job functions the job requires," observes Thorson. "But this ability varies from person to person with fibromyalgia. The problem is that people with FMS don't know how they're going to feel from day to day. There are times when they can work very competently, but then there are other times when they just can't go to work because they are in a pain flare. These people become undependable. This is disabling. They can't know if they can consistently work from 9 to 5 every day. They may be able to work 8:00 to 3:00 one day and then noon to midnight the next, but it's not consistent.

This job change has changed the course of Angie's fibromyalgia. She now has more time to focus on her own well-being.

"FMS also affects the ability to do lots of things," Thorson adds. "It might affect concentration and the ability to do cognitive tasks. The doctors who examine a patient before a disability hearing typically look at range of motion and ability to lift certain weights. They don't look at the person's ability to show up consistently at work."

Certainly, fibromyalgia does not fit into a neat category of disability, but no one involved in the treatment of FMS or committed to the support of people with FMS recommend long-term disability if it can be avoided. Dr. Turk offers his personal opinion: "Since most of us spend much of our time at work, it's not only where we earn our money, it's also where we have social contacts. It's a great part of our lives. I think that from the standpoint of self-esteem, to the extent that you're able to be out of the house doing something productive, I think it is an advantage to do as much as is reasonable.

"That's why I don't like the concept of disability for people with fibromyalgia," Dr. Turk says. "Our whole goal in treating patients with fibromyalgia is to teach them to function better despite the fact that they may have some limitations. If you're receiving disability, you're confirming the belief that 'there is nothing I can do.' I'd rather take the perspective of learning how to function better; the more you can do, even with limitations, the better it is for you. The more you focus on the way you can't do the things you used to do and don't have the activities related to the job that you used to have, the more limited you become and the more depressed you may tend to become. Disability can become a self-fulfilling prophecy. I encourage being active to a reasonable degree even though it's difficult."

> *Fibromyalgia does not fit into a neat category of disability, but no one involved in the treatment of FMS or committed to the support of people with it recommend long-term disability if it can be avoided.*

Some people with fibromyalgia, however, have no other choice; the pain and fatigue are simply too intense—they cannot work a full-time job. This seems to be the case with Raylene—the schoolteacher from Canada you met in chapter 3. When the pain and fatigue that followed each day of teaching a classroom full of energetic 6- and 7-year-olds became overwhelming, Raylene applied for disability, but the process itself has been very painful. After being diagnosed with fibromyalgia and spending weeks at a time in the hospital for painful muscle spasms in her back and legs, Raylene was told by her insurance company that before she could go on disability pay, she had to use up all her sick days, go to a psychologist, consult with a sports medicine specialist, and send in records from all her health care providers. After completing all the requirements, Raylene was granted half-day disability.

While she was working part-time, Raylene was required to attend physiotherapy twice a week to bounce on a ball, pull on rubber strings, ride stationary bikes, and the like. She would not receive her disability payment if she missed a session. Quite predictably, the physical stress of these treatments (which were not professionally tailored for fibromyalgia) and the hour drive to get to the facility were making all her symptoms worse.

Every week, Raylene was harassed with phone calls pushing her to return to work full-time. Rehabilitation specialists came to her workplace and embarrassed her in front of her colleagues. They wanted her to rest every 15 minutes (not easy to do when you're teaching!). "Every week they wanted to know when I'd be going back full-time. They just wouldn't let up."

Raylene went before an insurance board of 10 people to defend her case. "They looked at me and rolled their eyes as if to say, 'Yeah, right. You look fine to me.' They just couldn't get it that fibromyalgia isn't something you can see or that goes away." Finally, in tears, tired of being harassed, and feeling that the stress of fighting for a half-day of disability was making her symptoms worse, Raylene went back to work full-time.

> *Quite predictably, the physical stress of these treatments (which were not professionally tailored for fibromyalgia) and the hour drive to get to the facility were making all Raylene's symptoms worse.*

A few months later, Raylene was hospitalized for 8 days after another bout of muscle spasms. She returned home for 1 month and then went back to teaching part-time. "I can no longer go on like this," she cries. "I'm going to try to claim disability again because I have only 10 days' sick leave left, and I also will need future financial assistance if I can work only part-time. But I'm not looking forward to the harassment I experienced last time, so I'm thinking of getting a lawyer right away and letting him do all the fighting because I'm in no shape to handle the burden."

Sadly, Raylene's experience is not uncommon. The stress of fighting for disability pay can so badly worsen the symptoms of fibromyalgia that many medical professionals adamantly advise against it. Evidence indicates that the adversarial process of winning and maintaining a disability claim keeps the stress level so continuously high that the symptoms of FMS remain in a flare state without hope of relief.

"If You Have to Prove You Are Ill, You Can't Get Well" is the title of an editorial in the journal *Spine*, in which N. M. Hadler uses fibromyalgia as an object lesson. He points out that the legal process forces the person with fibromyalgia to demonstrate continually the magnitude of illness. "The litigant is likely to lose the prerequisite skills for well-being, the abilities to discern among the morbidities, and to cope. . . . Inexorably, the litigant is drawn into the vulnerable state, too often never to return," Hadler observes.[2]

> *Evidence indicates that the adversarial process of winning and maintaining a disability claim keeps the stress level so continuously high that the symptoms of FMS remain in a flare state without hope of relief.*

Despite the difficulties involved in filing claims and receiving awards, according to a 1997 study by Frederick Wolfe and colleagues, high rates of lifetime work disability payments are received by people with fibromyalgia across the country. In this study of 1,604 patients with FMS from six rheumatology centers (in Boston; Peoria, Illinois; Los Angeles; Portland, Oregon; San Antonio, Texas; and Wichita, Kansas), the average age of participants was 48.1 years, and 88.8 percent were female. When all sources (including Social Security, public assistance, and workers' compensation) were considered, 26.5 percent of all participants reported receiving a disability payment. The most important indicator of long-term disability is Social Security Disability (SSD) payments; 16.2 percent of patients with FMS reported such payments; by contrast, only 2.2 percent of adults living in those states received such payments.

These numbers do seem to label fibromyalgia as a disabling disease, but the other side of the issue—the *ability* to work—was also noted in this study. About two-thirds of all participants (64.3 percent), including 60.5 percent of homemakers, 68 percent of nonhomemakers, and 89.3 percent of those employed, reported being able to work most or all days. Only 19.4 percent stated they could work few or no days.[3] Obviously, FMS is not easily compartmentalized. It is as unique as each individual who is diagnosed.

Filing for Disability Benefits

It's true that Social Security Disability benefits can be difficult to receive if you do not have a visible disability (paralysis, blindness, etc.). Both SSD and long-term disability insurance carriers are exceptionally reluctant to pay out for illnesses that cannot be "proven." There are no x rays or blood tests to back up your claim. If you decide that you cannot work and need SSD support, you will have to go through a lengthy and tedious process of applications, hearings, and appeals. You will most likely have to hire an attorney, and you will wait many months, if not years, for a final ruling.

However, if you're up to fighting for what is rightfully yours, you have good news in your corner. In April 1999, the Social Security Administration issued new regulations that have caused a major setback to the judges, insurance companies, and expert medical witness who flat-out refuse to acknowledge FMS as a debilitating disease (or even a disease at all). Social Security Ruling 99-2p (referred to as SSR-99-2p) boldly announced that both fibromyalgia and chronic fatigue syndrome "are medically determinable conditions." This declaration legitimizes the clinical diagnosis and allows these syndromes to result in a finding of disability.

As hopeful as this ruling is, it does not mean that the diagnosis of FMS is automatically grounds to win a disability claim. You must first prove that you are "unable to engage in any substantial gainful activity due to a medically determinable mental or physical impairment, which has lasted or is expected to last at least 12 months or result in death, diagnosed by the patient's primary care or treating physician."[4]

Alec G. Sohmer, a lawyer from Brockton, Massachusetts, has built his practice on supporting the legal needs of people with fibromyalgia. He knows this can be a long and difficult process, but he also feels that with the proper legal help, those who are truly disabled by this chronic condition will eventually receive the disability payments they deserve.

Sohmer advises:

> *This can be a long and difficult process, but with the proper legal help, those who are truly disabled by this chronic condition will eventually receive the disability payments they deserve.*

The first step in determining your eligibility is to complete and file a written application at your local Social Security Office. Because considerable information is required to complete this form, you should visit or call the office beforehand to determine what supporting documentation is required.

Because fibromyalgia is not listed as a disabling condition on the list approved by the Social Security Office, expect a claim rejection. The listed impairments are specifically described physical or mental conditions that are so severe that the Social Security Administration has determined that persons suffering from those impairments are considered disabled. If your claim is rejected, you should appeal because benefits will be awarded if it is found that your condition causes substantially the same degree of functional limitations as other conditions on the approved list.

After receiving the initial rejection, you must then file for reconsideration. The request for reconsideration is the first step in the appellate process, which is also completed by application. (It is helpful to retain a copy of the initial application because the request for reconsideration seeks substantially the same information. This will reduce the time necessary to complete the second.)

If the reconsideration is denied, you must then file for administrative appeal. This step is where most fibromyalgia claimants are successful. The administrative judge must determine whether your condition causes the same degree of functional limitations as those listed. In determining what is a severe impairment, the administrative judge will consider any condition which significantly limits a claimant's ability to do basic work activities, such as walking, standing, lifting, bending, understanding, remembering, using judgment, and so on. The judge's decision will be based on medical evidence alone, which is lacking in fibromyalgia, so you will need to present a carefully documented case history. If properly presented, you are likely to succeed at this stage. Unfortunately, the entire process can take 2 years from start to finish.

Although the process may be lengthy, as many as 2 years from start to finish, Sohmer offers these tips to reduce the delay:

- Get started now.

- Prepare a list of each and every physician seen. This list should include names, phone numbers, addresses, approximate dates of treatment, and probable diagnoses. Remember to include all physicians, whether or not related to fibromyalgia.

> **Learn More**
> You can find more information about disability on Alec Sohmer's Web site:
>
> www.disabilityassistance
> .com

- Keep documents of medical records and how the condition affects your functional capacity on a daily basis.

- Talk to an experienced attorney who understands both the condition and Social Security laws.

"Hopefully," says Sohmer, "your fibromyalgia won't be so debilitating that you will need to seek retribution, but in the event that it is, you should persist until you get the benefits to which you are legally entitled."

Referral Resource

If you need a lawyer in your area to represent you in a disability claim, you might begin your search with a call to an organization called National Organization for Social Security Claimant Representatives (NOSSCR). This is a group of lawyers who do nothing but Social Security disability claims for any condition. They follow specific guidelines and charge fees (which are generally collected only if they win the case). Contact them at (800) 431-2804.

NURTURING YOUR RELATIONSHIP WITH YOURSELF

The most important relationship of all is the one you have with yourself. How do you feel about yourself? How do you treat yourself? How do you get along with yourself? The easiest way to evaluate this relationship is to listen to the conversations you have with yourself in your head and keep track of how many times you complain about your limitations, blame yourself for the problems caused by FMS, or heap on the guilt. As explained in chapter 5, more than other any daily communication, what you say to yourself will determine how you will live with fibromyalgia.

Fibromyalgia Is Not Who You Are

Thirty-five year-old Debby, who is a public relations/communications director for an e-business marketing company, was diagnosed with fibromyalgia about 5 years ago. The severity of Debby's symptoms covers a wide range. "It's a very inconsistently chronic problem in terms of the pain," says Debby. "The majority of my pain is in the neck, shoulders, and back area, but I also have pain in my chest almost daily (I've even gone to the hospital thinking it was a heart attack). Some days I can almost forget I have this problem, and other days, I will stand up from a sitting position and suddenly find that I literally can't move. This can wipe me out completely for the next 3 days. The scary thing for me is that this usually comes out of nowhere, so it's hard to prepare for it or make my plans around it."

Like anyone dealing with any kind of chronic condition, Debby knows having fibromyalgia affects her relationships. She feels that the one that has been most affected by fibromyalgia is the relationship she has with herself. "You go through life," says Debby, "thinking your life is going to be a certain way, and then you find out that you're not going to be who you thought you would be. I now have limits on what I can do that I have to deal with and build my life around. This change in the way I see myself—in the way I define who I am—is important to how all my other relationships work."

"For a while," admits Debby, "I let fibromyalgia be a part of who I was. As I got to know someone or if I went on a job interview, I felt obliged to explain that I had this condition. I spent a part of every day thinking about fibromyalgia and about how unfair it was that I had to have this illness that nobody else even heard of. But then the more I learned about fibromyalgia and came to accept that it's not going to go away, I knew I was going to have to find a better way to live with it. That's when I made a conscious effort not to make this disease be who I am. Now I personally refuse to spend my time, energy, or a single breath talking about fibromyalgia, unless it is to help other people who have it, too. This keeps me from letting fibromyalgia take over. I've learned that if I don't spend my day thinking about how unfair this is, I don't give myself as much to get depressed about. I've decided that I will not focus on this; I will not internalize it; I will not let myself get depressed about this. I just will not. This

> *I personally refuse to spend my time, energy, or a single breath talking about fibromyalgia, unless it is to help other people who have it, too.*
>
> —DEBBY

isn't denial—I know I have fibromyalgia and I will live with it, but I also know that if I keep busy thinking about other things, I can do more and live better. The relationship I have with myself is the most important relationship I have, and I have control over that."

When Debby reads about people who are completely disabled by fibromyalgia, she wonders whether maybe these people really do have more pain, fatigue, and other problems than she does or whether it may be a matter of how a person chooses to deal with this very difficult condition.

"Some days," she says, "I just can't go to work, and there's nothing I can do about that, but other days I'll wake up feeling just awful, and I just refuse to let that be the reason I fall back into bed and stay there. I've gone to work many times when I've been in terrible pain, and I've had to explain to my boss what's going on because sometimes I need him to understand why it might look like I'm not doing my best work. But I will not make it everyone else's issue. I've decided not to talk to any of my colleagues about this. I won't moan or complain. That's just not how I want to be defined by the people around me.

"I'm proud of the fact that I have decided that fibromyalgia will not control what I can and cannot do or ruin my life. I have made a conscious decision to live with this pain that can be very bad, but I will not let it take over my life. It is not who I am."

SUPPORT GROUPS

Support groups have given many people with fibromyalgia a lifeline when they thought they would surely drown. They can be an invaluable source of encouragement, information, and, of course, support that provides a better foundation on which to build all other relationships. They can also provide that understanding nod that a person who does not have fibromyalgia could never offer. No matter how supportive your family may be, only someone who has FMS can reassure you with the words "I know just what you mean." It's one thing, for example, to hear from a professional that you need to exercise or that you should get a good night's sleep, but it's another thing to hear from someone who also has fibromyalgia how she's struggling like you to implement this advice. It's fine for a counselor to say, "You have to learn how to ask for what you need," but it's additionally helpful to hear firsthand stories about how someone in your same situation has tried that. Knowing that you are not alone with your struggles can make life so much more bearable.

Support groups also offer a place for gathering information. Many discuss conventional and alternative treatments and trade experiences about what works and what doesn't. Some focus on learning new coping skills, such as relaxation exercises, cognitive restructuring, and daily exercise. And almost all leave time for exchanging tips on sleep, adaptive devices, travel, family, and work.

> *S*upport groups can be an invaluable source of encouragement, information, and, of course, support that provides a better foundation on which to build all other relationships.

For all the good that a support group can offer, it's surprising how many people with fibromyalgia avoid them. Echoing the fear of many, Rose, a 32-year-old computer programmer, says, "I tried going to a support group, and I hated it. It made me feel worse. I would sit and listen to everybody complaining, and I found myself joining in. I was spending more time than I ever wanted to talking about something that I really don't want to focus on. I want to find a way to live well with this condition and not spend so much time venting so much anger and frustration. I guess it's good to vent, but then you've got to get on with it. I'll never go to a support group again."

Kate Lorig, R.N., Dr.P.H., who is an associate professor in the Department of Medicine at Stanford University in California and author of *The Arthritis and Fibromyalgia Helpbook* (Perseus Publishing, 2000), understands why people like Rose avoid support groups. Lorig is presently involved in moderating and evaluating the effects of a

2-year-old online support group for 250 people with chronic back pain. She feels that some people have bad experiences with support groups for three primary reasons:

- **The group does not have a moderator.** To be a positive, worthwhile effort, a support group has to have a good moderator who can keep the talk moving in a positive direction. Support groups without a strong leader can quickly turn into pity parties. Unless they are really well led, you sit and listen to one horror story after another as people play a game called "my disease is worse than your disease." Good moderators are often health professionals such as a medical doctor, a psychologist, or a physical therapist, but not always. Many groups are led by lay people who do an excellent job. Whoever is moderating has to keep the group from turning the meeting into a gripe session.

- **You may misunderstand the purpose of a support group.** Some people find themselves involved with a very good group but feel let down because they were hoping for more time to complain and share their misery. A good leader may say, "I understand that you all have had bad experiences, but I want to talk about what you are going to do this week to make things better." Well, that leaves no time for whining, does it? This is more of a challenge than an offer of sympathy, so when this happens, some participants who were expecting more hand holding leave very discouraged.

- **The sponsoring organization may misunderstand the purpose of a support group.** Sometimes support groups sponsored by health organizations are really more of a lecture program. They are called "support groups" because people do get together and talk a little bit, but the focus of the gathering is a lecture on a health-related issue. This approach, too, can be very helpful—if that's what you want. But if you expect a give-

and-take experience and end up in a lecture situation, you could easily get turned off to the idea of support groups completely.

If you try an online support group, chat room, or e-mail discussion group, Lorig advises caution. With neither ground rules nor a moderator, you may quickly find that you've fallen in with a group of angry complainers. This is especially true online because here people will say things they would never say face to face. Look for words of encouragement rather than blame. Look for objective and helpful input over personalized tantrums. Look for constructive "to-do" advice rather than "I-can't-do" testimonials. Spend some time surfing through these sites, and choose carefully the ones you would like to join.

> *With neither ground rules nor a moderator, you may quickly find that you've fallen in with a group of angry complainers.*

To find a good support group, Lorig suggests that you contact a reputable organization and ask for a referral. You might try the Arthritis Foundation or the Fibromyalgia Network (see the appendix for details). You might also ask your doctor whether he or she knows of a local group or ask a representative from your health plan if they are sponsoring anything.

LIVING WELL WITH FIBROMYALGIA

Penney Cowan of the American Chronic Pain Association has had a very personal experience with fibromyalgia that gives her words of encouragement added weight. As you think about how your fibromyalgia affects your relationships at home, with your kids, at work, and with yourself, keep her words in mind: "I think people need to know that you can have a full life in spite of pain. When I first enrolled in a pain program for fibromyalgia 21 years ago, I really thought my life was at the very end. I went there with every intention of failing because I did not believe that anything in the world could

Tips for Evaluating FMS Support Groups

- Make sure the group has a strong moderator.

- Stay away from groups that allow participants to spend the majority of time complaining.

- Look for a group that will give you resources and information.

- Find a group that will motivate you to help yourself.

- Stick with a group that supports and applauds your efforts.

ever help me. And I had absolutely no ability to help myself. I thought medicine was supposed to fix me. It never occurred to me that I had to be a part of my own treatment team.

"But that's where it's at," Cowan says. "The person with fibromyalgia has to be actively involved in living well, and we all have to accept responsibility for the quality of life we live."

CHAPTER 8

Fibromyalgia and the Future

THROUGHOUT THE PAGES of this book, you have found answers to many of the riddles associated with fibromyalgia, but many questions remain. You may be left wondering, "What caused my fibromyalgia?" "Will I pass this on to my children?" "Why are some people more severely affected than others?" "Why does a particular treatment plan work so well for one person with fibromyalgia and utterly fail for another?" "Why do so many doctors pretend fibromyalgia doesn't exist?" As you consider these and other important questions, you'll be happy to hear that medical investigators and others in the health care profession are now asking them as well. Finally, fibromyalgia is beginning to receive the attention and funding necessary to unlock these mysteries and offer you new hope for more effective treatment in the near future.

A LOOK BACK

I. Jon Russell, M.D., Ph.D., of the University of Texas Health Sciences Center in San Antonio, is a true pioneer in the field of fibro-

Strength in Numbers

Epidemiology is the study of populations to determine how common certain medical conditions are. The epidemiologic study of fibromyalgia has revealed some surprising facts. Its occurrence rate in the U.S. general population is about 2 percent of all adults (over five million affected persons and 3.2 percent of all females). The occurrence rate increases with age, until it is found in about 10 percent of women 50 to 60 years of age.[1] As these studies determine that more people have fibromyalgia than originally thought, this disorder becomes more scientifically established as a condition that deserves medical and even political attention.

myalgia research. He began working in this area of medicine in 1980 (when it was known as fibrositis) and began to conduct research on this subject long before the American College of Rheumatology published the standards of diagnostic criteria in 1990 that validated the existence of this syndrome. Throughout these years, he has attained international recognition for his hard work and unfailing dedication to fibromyalgia research. It is because of Dr. Russell and a handful of others like him that this book could be written, that there is an improved understanding of this disorder, and that millions like you will someday soon be able to say, "I have fibromyalgia," without receiving stares of surprise as if you just said, "I have three heads."

Dr. Russell's experiences in the field of fibromyalgia will give you an idea of how far we have come in a relatively short time:

Because I came to the field with a doctorate degree in biochemistry in addition to my doctorate in medicine, my colleagues anticipated that I would study some very basic science topic, perhaps confining myself to the chemistry laboratory. But I saw these patients who were struggling with pain and who were frustrated by the way they were treated by their physicians and other health care workers like physical therapists, psychologists, and others. Of course, they were doubting themselves and wondering if they weren't going crazy. I felt the challenge to tackle this area and found myself waging an uphill battle. We had no idea what to do or where to begin such a study, and there was also the problem of peer resistance.

The number of investigators working with fibromyalgia was limited to those who were stubborn enough and sufficiently motivated to persist in spite of the obstacles and ridicule. For example, one day I was told by one of my chairmen at the medical school that I would never be promoted academically if I continued to work on 'fibrositis.' This was very threatening to me as a young faculty member because the two important goals of my life work were to learn new things that could help my patients and to eventually earn the respect of my peers. It seemed clear that the latter wasn't going to happen.

On another occasion, I was asked by my chairman to head up the education component of a multipurpose arthritis center grant proposal. I asked him if I could propose a fibromyalgia study; he said no way would he allow me to place the institution and the overall project at risk by including a fibromyalgia grant. This kind of negative pressure has no doubt inhibited fibromyalgia research in the past, but I felt that this condition needed investigation and had the potential to make progress, so I persisted.

> *The number of investigators working with fibromyalgia was limited to those who were stubborn enough and sufficiently motivated to persist in spite of the obstacles and ridicule.*
>
> —I. JON RUSSELL, M.D., PH.D.

It is because of the persistence of researchers like Dr. Russell that so many good things are happening today in the study of fibromyalgia. "Sometimes I have to pinch myself when I think about what has happened over the last 20 years of research in this area," says Dr. Russell. "It's unbelievable to me that I have had the opportunity to discover things that were not known before and to be involved in the process of taking a disorder which was largely ignored and considered a waste of research time to the point of learning things that are actually quite remarkable.

"I am very encouraged by the new ideas and energetic new talent that has been attracted to this field in the last decade. If I can be so brave as to predict the future based upon events of recent past, I would forecast a dramatic increase in our knowledge about the causes of fibromyalgia and unprecedented progress in the development of safe and effective methods of treatment for its symptoms."

WHAT TO EXPECT FROM THE PEOPLE INVOLVED IN THE FIELD

Who are the people who will drive the expected changes in the field of fibromyalgia research and treatment? They are physicians, scientific investigators, pharmaceutical companies, health insurance companies, and those who belong to support organizations—all in addition to the millions who have fibromyalgia and persistently push for answers.

Physicians

Rae Gleason, an activist associated with the National Fibromyalgia Research Association in Salem, Oregon, has seen awareness and concern among physicians steadily grow in recent years. "When I first started going to the American Academy of Family Physicians meeting in 1994," she says, "these doctors shunned our booth and walked right by. The next year, a few stopped and asked for information, the next year a few more, and now they are standing in line waiting for the new information we have to give them. More and more physicians are now desperately trying to find help for their patients who have been diagnosed with FMS."

This is a very positive sign. It increases the likelihood of a correct diagnosis and a more focused treatment plan—which was not so likely to happen in the past. Gleason says that she now realizes that her own mother had fibromyalgia but was never diagnosed:

> She had the leg jerks at night; she had irritable bowel syndrome, heightened sensitivity to pain, and widespread pain. I remember that she would call me into her bedroom in the morning to help her lift her arms off the bed because they hurt so badly. I would go with her to the doctor, and he would say, "You have a little arthritis, but nothing that should be hurting you that badly." I sat and heard doctors say all the things that people tell me today doctors have said to them, and I realize now what was going on. My mother eventually ended up in a nursing home with Parkinson's disease, and so often when I'd ask her how she was doing, she'd say, "Oh, I'm just fine if I just didn't hurt all over." I know that if she went to a doctor with these symptoms today, there's a good possibility that she would be diagnosed with fibromyalgia and treated for these symptoms.

It may be too late for Gleason's mother, but still this activist-daughter is optimistic. "I look at this as an exciting time for fibromyalgia," Gleason says. "We've come a long way in the last 10 years. We have a long way to go, but we've opened up a lot of doors. From the beginning of time people have been suffering with fibromyalgia with no answers at all. Now we're on the threshold of having many answers. It will happen."

Gleason's observations about the changing attitudes in the medical profession are right on target. As scientific research uncovers the biological factors involved in fibromyalgia, medical school instructors will have more courage and more reasons to teach their students about these mechanisms. Dr. Russell believes, "As future doctors learn about the newly understood mechanisms, they obviously are going to be learning about fibromyalgia as the best clinical example of those abnormalities in pain perception. So when they go out into practice, their first fibromyalgia patient will not be a shock to them." This itself is a great step forward.

This change in the way fibromyalgia is recognized and diagnosed by physicians may have more positive ramifications than the much-welcomed respect for the dignity of each patient. The pain literature shows that people who have pain for a short period of time are more likely to recover completely if the treatment is right than are those who have a similar amount of pain but have had it for many years; in those cases, the chronic aspect of the pain is locked in. Understanding FMS, recognizing it earlier in its course, and treating it properly may actually prevent the transition into a chronic pain state.

*A*s scientific research uncovers the biological factors involved in fibromyalgia, medical school instructors will have more courage and more reasons to teach their students about these mechanisms.

Investigators

The number of people involved in the field of fibromyalgia has increased dramatically over the last 10 years. With great enthusiasm, Dr. Russell predicts that "an increasing number of young investigators will see fibromyalgia as the opportunity of a lifetime and they will make it their life's work. They are going to bring to the field wonderful new talents, enthusiasm, energy, and skills to study this problem."

This optimistic prediction is based on what Dr. Russell has seen since 1990 when he and others at the American College of Rheumatology published the diagnostic criteria for fibromyalgia. "During the 1970s and 1980s," remembers Dr. Russell, "about 10 to 15 research papers were published on the subject of fibromyalgia every year. But then around 1990, the number of annual publications on this subject shot up to about 120 and has stayed up at that level ever since. This nearly tenfold increase in published papers on FMS represents a dramatic increase attributable directly to the validation of diagnostic criteria."

This validation also means that a public sponsoring agency such as the National Institutes of Health (NIH) could conscientiously spend some of the country's money studying the disorder because it could be identified in a reproducible way. Dr. Russell continues:

The Fibromyalgia Network organization, led by Kristin Thorson, sponsored my testimony to the U.S. Congress and House of Representatives budget committees in 1994 about the need for fibromyalgia education and research funding. At that time, the amount of federal funding for fibromyalgia annually was only about $200,000 for the work of a single investigator. I was gratified that the next year the NIH announced a call for proposals to study fibromyalgia and that about 45 researchers responded. That number represented substantially more investigators than were known to be interested in fibromyalgia before that date.

The NIH's willingness to fund fibromyalgia research had attracted to the field new people with their unique ideas, talents, and skills. The NIH funded five of those new investigators. It was very clear that funding made it possible for investigators who had not studied fibromyalgia before to swallow their pride, to buck the establishment, and to submit a fibromyalgia grant proposal. That was a very exciting new development. It meant that the numbers of disciplines involved in the study of fibromyalgia was going to expand and that new approaches to studying the disorder would be proposed. It meant that the resources of many new institutions would be involved in the process of studying fibromyalgia. The young investigators would be working with more sophistication in their research methods and with less risk of peer ridicule.

Because fibromyalgia syndrome is a very common medical problem in the general population, and because fibromyalgia patients are usually quite willing to participate in research studies, these new investigators would have adequate numbers of subjects to study. I think this was the most encouraging and hopeful news I had seen in the last 10 years.

Pharmaceutical Companies

The fact that the NIH is now recognizing fibromyalgia as a real disorder and that the epidemiology studies around the world say that this disorder is more common than rheumatoid arthritis (somewhere between two and five times as common) gives pharmaceutical companies reasons to invest in research on this disorder. Here is a new market for them.

"A number of pharmaceutical companies are coming to me and to other investigators and saying, 'How can we study fibromyalgia? It looks like there is a huge market for this.'" says Dr. Russell. "I have tried to encourage these companies to invest research dollars to find medications that target the specific biological abnormalities that we have found are associated with fibromyalgia. Most of these abnormalities focus on the central nervous system, and they suggest impairment of the central nervous system process of pain perception. If that is the case, we now have a target for biochemical research. That is the kind of thing that intrigues drug companies." Dr. Russell feels certain that we are on the threshold of major research investments by pharmaceutical companies on the causes of fibromyalgia and on medications that will specifically target its symptoms.

Health Insurance Companies

Health insurance agencies have been very skeptical and very afraid of fibromyalgia. In the past, most have been successful in ignoring it and have found ways to drop people who develop fibromyalgia by saying that it is a psychiatric problem (which they generally don't cover). What is needed and foreseeable in the future is a way to document pain. We have x rays for broken bones, imaging studies for gallstones and tumors, endoscopy for ulcers, and magnetic resonance imaging (MRI) for brain structures, but we don't yet have a way to measure pain that would concretely validate the existence of fibromyalgia.

> *We are on the threshold of major research investments by pharmaceutical companies on the causes of fibromyalgia and on medications that will specifically target its symptoms.*

"I'm hoping that the studies involving fibromyalgia will lead the way to finding objective measures of pain," says Dr. Russell. "When medical technology can actually measure pain and document its intensity, then there will be a mandate to be more fair with people who experience pain. The same technology will be used to identify treatments that are effective in safely relieving the pain. Pain conditions will be viewed in the same light as a broken bone or blood dripping from a damaged vessel. Insurance companies will have the objective basis they have needed to more accurately forecast fiduciary risk and will voluntarily include pain conditions into their policies to support people with fibromyalgia. This will be a tremendous contribution to this field that will spread out into many other areas of health care."

Support Organizations

Numerous fibromyalgia support organizations have been established over the last decade (see the appendix for a partial listing). These groups have been and will continue to be a force to increase public awareness of the needs of people with fibromyalgia. Some fibromyalgia support organizations raise funds to sponsor research, some pressure legislators to allocate federal research funds, some provide information and support those who have fibromyalgia, and others have been instrumental in pressuring the U.S. government to pay attention to fibromyalgia. There's no doubt that in the future these groups will grow (despite the inevitable ego problems and competition that will pit some against others), and they will maintain the momentum for allocating provisions for fibromyalgia patients.

WHAT TO EXPECT FROM RESEARCH

It's quite clear that research investigators have made impressive strides in understanding fibromyalgia from both a clinical and biological viewpoint. Following is a sampling of some of the research that has been and is continuing to be conducted in the search for a cause and a cure:

- **I. Jon Russell, M.D., Ph.D.,** of the University of Texas Health Sciences Center in San Antonio, and his colleagues are continuing their study of the elevated level of the neurotransmitter substance P (which the body's pain neurons normally release into the spinal cord when peripheral tissues are injured) that is found to be elevated in the spinal fluid of most patients with fibromyalgia.

- **Daniel Clauw, M.D.,** of Georgetown University, is conducting a study to demonstrate that pain sensitivity is an independent trait determined primarily by physiological factors (e.g., neurotransmitters in cerebrospinal fluid), and not a surrogate for psychological factors such as depression, anxiety, or work-related stressors.

- **Roland Staud, M.D.,** of the University of Florida, has found ample evidence showing that fibromyalgia patients have an abnormal central nervous system pain mechanism, or pain memory, that results in sensations that linger much longer than usual and require much less stimulation to activate them.

- **Laurence Bradley, Ph.D.,** of the University of Alabama, is conducting a study to better understand the mechanisms responsible for inhibited functional brain activity observed in FMS patients during rest.

- **Peter Rowe, M.D.,** a pediatric cardiologist at Johns Hopkins University, has conducted studies that find that about 30 percent of FMS patients suffer from neurally mediated hypotension (NMH) and that administration of low blood pressure medications and increases in salt intake can dramatically reduce the severity of their symptoms.

- **Robert Bennett, M.D.,** of the Oregon Health Science University, has demonstrated that some FMS patients have abnormally low levels of growth hormone. He has also found that approximately one-third of people with fibromyalgia developed fibromyalgia after having some kind of trauma.

- **Leslie Crofford, M.D.,** of the University of Michigan, Ann Arbor, is researching abnormal growth hormone and cortisol levels in FMS patients.

- **Muhammad Yunus, M.D.,** of the University of Illinois at Peoria, and **Jane Olson, Ph.D.,** of Case Western Reserve University in Ohio, are conducting separate studies of the genetic component of fibromyalgia.

- **Garth L. Nicolson, Ph.D.,** and colleagues present a compelling case arguing that the disorders chronic fatigue syndrome (CFS), fibromyalgia, Gulf War illness (GWI), and a number of other chronic illnesses stem from a similar cause—infection by a primitive bacterium called a *mycoplasm*.

- Neurosurgeons **Michael Rosner, M.D.,** of the University of Alabama in Birmingham, and **Dan S. Heffez, M.D.,** of the Chicago Institute of Neurosurgery and Neuroresearch, have found that some people with fibromyalgia also have another type of clinical problem called *Chiari syndrome* or *cervical spinal stenosis*—a narrowing of the opening at the base of the skull or in the neck that compresses the lower part of the brain or spinal cord.

WHAT TO EXPECT IN TREATMENT

The sampling of current research projects just provided is certainly encouraging, but it brings up a sticking point. As with all other disorders, effective treatment of fibromyalgia is dependent on researchers' ability to pinpoint its cause. But you'll notice that many of the researchers are looking for the cause of FMS in very diverse places. Some think FMS is caused by dysfunctional hormone production; others say it's caused by primitive bacteria; still others are looking into dysfunctions in the central nervous system, and on and on. Naturally, the big question is, "Who's right?"

Long-Term Follow-Up

In the longest follow-up study from a single medical center, 29 patients with FMS were surveyed, 1, 3, and 14 years after diagnosis. Although 16 (55 percent) of 29 patients still reported moderate to severe pain, fatigue, and sleep disturbances, 19 (66 percent) of 29 felt better than when first diagnosed 14 years earlier, and 16 (73 percent) of 29 thought that their symptoms interfered little, if at all, with their work.[2]

The answer to this very complex question is starting to take form. Remember that fibromyalgia is a syndrome, not a well-defined disease; therefore, it would not be far-fetched to find that they are all right—for different subgroups of people with chronic pain like fibromyalgia.

Dr. Russell explains: "At first we thought the label 'syndrome' would quickly make the transition to 'disease'. Now it appears more likely that fibromyalgia is not a single disorder but a combination of several disorders that have different causes and different perpetuating factors that our bodies have only a limited number of ways to deal with. I think we will find that fibromyalgia has a variety of causes."

He likens this possibility to what might happen with a hypothetical condition called the 'limping syndrome': A patient with the limping syndrome may be acting that way because his foot pain is caused by an unrecognized splinter, a stubbed toe, an ingrown toenail, or a fractured bone, but the end result is the same pattern of limping. If the doctor had no way of knowing the cause of the limping, he would diagnose "limping syndrome" and use his pet treatment—let's say rest and elevation. He would find that it helped most of the limpers somewhat and some of the limpers a great deal (e.g., those who have a hairline fracture). The limpers who did not benefit as much might be those who had an unrecognized splinter or ingrown toenail. The doctor might assume that those who did not respond to his treatment were either faking their symptoms or not properly complying with his treatment program. How frustrating for everyone involved! In this obvious case, we can see that prescribing the same treatment to all patients with "limping syndrome" makes no sense—even though they all come to the physician with the same symptom of limping. It now appears that this might be exactly what is happening with fibromyalgia.

> *R*emember that fibromyalgia is a syndrome, not a well-defined disease.

"The trouble with the diagnosis of fibromyalgia is that we may be putting people in this category who have similar symptoms but who in fact may have different mechanisms causing these symptoms," observes Dennis C. Turk, Ph.D., professor of anesthesiology and pain research at the University of Washington in Seattle. "In the literature on fibromyalgia, you'll see that when someone publishes a new treatment study, a statistically significant percentage of people with FMS (about 30 percent) report great benefit, and everyone becomes very excited. Then another, very different treatment comes along that also significantly helps about 30 percent of the people with fibromyalgia. Exercise, trigger point injections, psychotherapy, and the like, all end up helping about 30 percent of the people who try them. How can a disorder have these same outcomes with these very different treatments?"

Dr. Turk's work on fibromyalgia "subsets" proposes that we should be looking at fibromyalgia as being made up of different groups of people. Perhaps there are subgroups of people who, although they have a similar set of symptoms, may be quite different. "Maybe," he wonders, "the reason we see so many different treatments working on different people is that they don't all come to fibromyalgia from the same place."

This subset theory would also explain the dilemma of overlapping conditions associated with FMS. "We now recognize that fibromyalgia

FIBROMYALGIA AND THE FUTURE

is many different things to different parts of the body," says Dr. Russell. "We recognize and know statistically the prevalence with which people with fibromyalgia have pain, have limitation in function, have involvement of the bowel, have headaches, have pain with movement of the chest, have depression, have slightly elevated sedimentation rates, and have abnormalities in the antinuclear antibody. We will eventually develop the ability to understand individuals in each of these subcategories and see how their diverse presentations relate to the fibromyalgia syndrome. This allows the overlapping of symptoms to seem less mysterious and helps physicians to better understand their patients who exhibit variant patterns of symptoms. Soon physicians will be saying, 'Let's try to figure out the pattern of fibromyalgia in *you*.'"

> *The trouble with the diagnosis of fibromyalgia is that we may be putting people in this category who have similar symptoms but who in fact may have different mechanisms causing these symptoms.*
>
> —DENNIS C. TURK, PH.D.

Dr. Turk's research on subsets asks the following questions:

- Can we identify subgroups of patients based on how they respond to a common set of questions about their symptoms?

- On a statistical basis, is there a set of signs and symptoms that fit together in a meaningful way that we could then design a treatment for?

According to Dr. Turk, "This is very different from the present method that works on the premise, 'If I try enough stuff, I'll get some beneficial effect without ever really knowing why.' Right now we're treating people who have the diagnosis of fibromyalgia as if they were all the same—future research is going to show us that they are not. We're going to be able to categorize people with fibromyalgia by biochemical, endocrinological, and biomechanical factors and then statistically identify patterns of responding to pain that would indicate a particular treatment plan."

Dr. Turk is hoping to establish a way to match treatments to patients' unique characteristics. "Specifically, we will test the efficacy of uniquely tailored treatment for each psychosocial or biomedical subgroup, and establish the benefit of matching treatments to subject characteristics, and enhance our understanding of the roles of cognitive-affective-behavioral adaptation of FMS patients."

It now appears that receiving the diagnosis of "fibromyalgia" is only the beginning of the journey to wellness. "Originally we thought we would identify the cause of fibromyalgia and then progress to the disease status in our scientific investigation," admits Dr. Russell. "But now I can see that it's possible that this won't happen. That is not necessarily a bad thing; I see it as an advance because by finding different ideologies, we may in fact find different approaches to treatment, which in turn could reduce the incidence of fibromyalgia and improve the outcome of the disorder once it develops." This end result will be good news for everyone with fibromyalgia.

Team Treatment Centers

Pooling this knowledge about subsets and accepting the concept that people can come to the diagnosis of fibromyalgia from very different places would be a giant step toward finding effective treatment regimens—assuming the physicians from different disciplines can work together.

> *Accepting the concept that people can come to the diagnosis of fibromyalgia from very different places would be a giant step toward finding effective treatment regimens—assuming the physicians from different disciplines can work together.*

Many working in this field believe that in the ideal situation, fibromyalgia team treatment centers will exist in which health care providers from a variety of disciplines will pool their talents to give each person with fibromyalgia personalized diagnostic and treatment care.

Rae Gleason of the National Fibromyalgia Research Association remembers when Dr. Robert Bennett set up the first multidisciplinary fibromyalgia treatment program at the Oregon Health Sciences University in the late 1980s. "Along with Dr. Bennett," recalls Gleason, "Dr. Sharon Clark, an exercise physiologist, Dr. Carol Burckhardt, a psychologist, and a team of other professionals worked diligently with FMS patients to improve their physical and mental well-being. The program helped develop an exercise regimen and offered appropriate medications for sleep and pain and psychological counseling to help patients cope with life changes resulting from fibromyalgia. It was very successful, but the insurance companies wouldn't reimburse the real costs, so, unfortunately, it was eventually dismantled."

> *In the ideal situation, health care providers from a variety of disciplines will pool their talents to give each person with fibromyalgia personalized diagnostic and treatment care.*

Then rheumatologist Philip Mease, M.D., of Seattle helped develop such a multidisciplinary program for fibromyalgia, chronic fatigue syndrome, and chronic rheumatic diseases in the late 1980s; it is still up and running and serves as a model of what could be down the road for fibromyalgia care. "The synergy of a group of physical and occupational therapists, psychologic and vocational counselors, biofeedback specialists, acupuncturists, nurse educators, and physicians all working under one roof to customize the care of individuals has been beneficial for the patients and morale-boosting for the providers," said Dr. Mease in an interview reported in *Fibromyalgia Network Newsletter*. Sensing the value of treatment provided by a variety of disciplines, "the program grew from a need arising in the world of community practice, primarily for better patient care, but secondarily to prevent provider burnout."[3]

A team program offers many benefits. Each specialist gains additional education and support from other members, providers are better able to assess treatment outcomes, and a team approach can reduce overall cost of care by coordinating efforts. As for the patients, the program's value is derived from its ability to help them improve and better cope with their illness because it offers them access to a variety of highly qualified individual practitioners who listen to them, believe in them, and know how to treat them.

Dr. Gleason explains:

One of my dreams is to get insurance companies involved in innovative funding of a multidisciplinary clinic just for people with fibromyalgia.

It would staff a neurologist, a neurosurgeon, a rheumatologist, a psychologist, an exercise physiologist, a physical therapist, and a nutritionist. It would be a place where after diagnosis, the patient would be further tested to find out if the cause was based in neurology, rheumatology, endocrinology, and so on, and then treatment programs would be tailored to the illness. This program would then be accepted by family physicians who would then help their patients comply with the plan. That would be so successful for so many people.

The program's value is derived from its ability to help people improve and better cope with their illness because it offers them access to a variety of highly qualified individual practitioners who listen to them, believe in them, and know how to treat them.

To me, this seems better than dumping money down a hole funding treatments that are not helping fibromyalgia patients. Insurance money could be much better spent in a multidisciplinary fibromyalgia center to promote healing rather than ineffective treatment. Somebody has to start somewhere to find a way to better help people with this condition. This would be a very positive direction.

WHAT TO EXPECT TOMORROW

As knowledge increases, attitudes change. Think back 20 years ago. Did your school system worry about how children in wheelchairs would get into the building? Did anyone at a public meeting stop to consider that people with disabilities might not be able to navigate the staircase leading to the meeting room? Did anyone care where such people had to park their cars? Of course not. It took years of public

Growth of Information

A few years ago, a person who was lucky enough to find a doctor who could correctly diagnose fibromyalgia was then dropped into the empty pit of information darkness. There were no books written on the subject, no Internet sites to surf, and no support groups to reach out to. Today's vast supply of information is a very healthy sign that fibromyalgia has arrived as a disorder worthy of focus, time, and attention.

education, letter-writing campaigns, legislative hearings, organizational funding, and unrelenting persistence by advocates for the physically challenged to bring about a change in public awareness, then attitude, then law.

The same process is underway today for fibromyalgia. Few think about what you need to navigate through life with this condition. Few worry that you'll be able to continue working and support your family. Few even know that such a syndrome exists. But all that will change over the next few years as fibromyalgia advocates, investigators, organizations, and the voices of the millions of people with fibromyalgia speak out louder and more frequently.

Without a doubt, you'll see attitude changes that will make wishes come true. It is likely that the problems of people with FMS will be addressed by physicians who not only will lack the bias of prior generations against the disorder but will be knowledgeable about how to diagnose and treat it. People with FMS who wake with disabling morning stiffness will hopefully find that their employers are more understanding of their trouble with early mornings and will allow them to start work later in the day. Many more will work from home, where they can maintain their work function and still accommodate their physical needs. These changes will allow people with fibromyalgia to live up to their educational and financial potential more effectively. They will also be more likely get a fair hearing from insurance agencies and will be a prime marketing target for pharmaceutical companies. We can hope that someday, when people with FMS say, "I have fibromyalgia," the people they are talking to will say, "Oh, I have heard of that; what can I do to help you?"

> *Fibromyalgia advocates, investigators, organizations, and the voices of the millions of people with fibromyalgia speak out louder and more frequently.*

Does this kind of future sound like something you've dared to imagine, if only in a dream? Well, now you can begin to picture it as part of your future reality. Thanks to the hard work of determined and supportive research investigators and to the many individuals with FMS who feel empowered to work hard at finding a remedy that fits their needs (and when that fails to try another and another!), you have reason to hope that tomorrow will be much better than today.

Appendix: Resource Information

IN THIS AGE of instant information access, there are many resources that can help you gather the facts about fibromyalgia syndrome. The organizations, Web sites, books, and booklets printed here are recommended for your use. When searching for more information, you should beware, however, of false, misleading, and bogus information. In a paper presented to the 63rd Annual Scientific Meeting of The American College of Rheumatology in 1999, Daniel Goldenberg, M.D., offered these words of warning:

> In order to assess the sources, content and quality of medical information concerning fibromyalgia on the Internet, we searched all sites on the World Wide Web, using Yahoo, Excite and Lycos search engines. As of fall 1999 there were 120 sites on the Web dedicated to FM information. Sponsors of these Web sites were 55% patients with FM, 14% FM organizations, 9% government or medical school institutions and 9% commercial sites. Forty-six percent sold products, usually books, vitamins or alternative health care products. Nine percent of sites had religious information.
>
> We evaluated the quality of FM medical information by contrasting diagnostic, pathogenic and therapeutic recommendations of each site to that of peer-reviewed journals. Misinformation about FM was prominent, especially from

those sites sponsored by patients and by health care professionals. On those sites, greater than 50% of information about FM pathogenesis and treatment was inaccurate. The quality of medical information on FM found on the Web is often poor and affected by sponsor bias.

Keep this in mind as you search for new information about fibromyalgia syndrome.

SUPPORT ORGANIZATIONS

American Chronic Pain Association
P.O. Box 850
Rocklin, CA 95677
Phone: (916) 632-0922
E-mail: ACPA@pacbell.net
Web site: www.theacpa.org

American College of Rheumatology
1800 Century Place, Suite 250
Atlanta, GA 30345
Phone: (404) 633-3777
Fax: (404) 633-1870
E-mail: acr@rheumatology.org
Web site: www.rheumatology
   .org

American Fibromyalgia Syndrome Association, Inc. (AFSA)
6380 Tanque Verde, Suite D
Tucson, AZ 85715
Phone: (520) 733-1570
Web site: www.afsafund.org

Arthritis Foundation
1330 W. Peachtree Street
Atlanta, GA 30309

Phone: (800) 283-7800
Web site: www.arthritis.org

The Arthritis Foundation publishes the *Fibromyalgia Wellness Letter* six times a year with the latest research findings on FMS, tips on exercise and nutrition, mind-body techniques, and advice on coping.

Fibromyalgia Association— USA
P.O. Box 20408
Columbus, OH 43220
E-mail: FibroUSA@Fibro
   myalgiaassnusa.org
Web site: www.fibromyalgia
   assnusa.org

Fibromyalgia Network
P.O. Box 31750
Tucson, AZ 85751
Phone: (800) 853-2929
Web site: www.fmnetnews.com

Established 1987, this information resource now has over 30,000 subscribers. This site is provided for the purpose of assisting patients in understanding their condition.

International MyoPain Society
P. O. Box 690402
San Antonio, TX 78269
Phone: (210) 567-4661
Fax: (210) 567-6669
Web site: www.myopain.org

National Fibromyalgia Awareness Campaign
2415 N. River Trail Road, #200
Orange, CA 92865
Phone: (714) 921-0150
E-mail: nfac1@aol.com
Web site: www.fmaware.com

The National Fibromyalgia Research Association (NFRA)
P.O. Box 500
Salem, OR 97302
Web site: www.nfra.net

An activist organization.

National Institute of Arthritis, Musculoskeletal, and Skin Diseases
National Institutes of Health
9000 Rockville Pike
Bethesda, MD 20892
Web site: www.nih.gov/niams

Free packet of fibromyalgia information containing lists of fibromyalgia organizations, a glossary, the American College of Rheumatology's Fact Sheet, and several FMS articles written by experts.

National Organization for Social Security Claimant Representatives (NOSSCR)
6 Prospect Street
Midland Park, NJ 07432
Phone: (800) 431-2804
E-mail: nosscr@worldnet.att.net
Web site: www.nosscr.org

This is a group of lawyers who do nothing but SS disability claims for any condition. They have guidelines they follow and fees they charge (which are generally collected if they win the case).

The Oregon Fibromyalgia Foundation (OFF)
Web site: www.myalgia.com

This site, written and maintained by researcher Robert M. Bennett, M.D., has articles on FMS.

BOOKS

Fibromyalgia: A Comprehensive Approach: What You Can Do About Chronic Pain and Fatigue by Miryam Ehrlich Williamson and David A. Nye (Walker & Co., 1996).

The Fibromyalgia Help Book: Practical Guide to Living Better With Fibromyalgia by Jenny Fransen and I. Jon Russell (Smith House, 1997).

The Fibromyalgia Relief Book: 213 Ideas for Improving Your Quality of Life by Miryam Ehrlich Williamson and Mary Anne Saathoff (Walker & Co., 1998).

BOOKLETS

Fibromyalgia Syndrome: An Informational Guide for FMS Patients and their Families by Robert Bennett, M.D. Order from: National Fibromyalgia Research Association, P.O. Box 500, Salem, OR 97302.

Fibromyalgia Syndrome and Chronic Fatigue Syndrome in Young People: A Guide For Parents by Kristin Thorson, Health Information Network, Inc. Order from: Fibromyalgia Network, P.O. Box 31750, Tucson, AZ 85751; (800) 853-2929.

Getting the Most Out of Your Medicines. Order from: Fibromyalgia Network, P.O. Box 31750, Tucson, AZ 85751; (800) 853-2929.

Notes

Chapter 1

1. "Fibromyalgia Syndrome: A Patient's Guide," The Fibromyalgia Network, January 2001.
2. M.B. Yunus, "Fibromyalgia Syndrome and Myofascial Pain Syndrome: Clinical Features, Laboratory Tests, Diagnosis, and Pathophysiologic Mechanisms," in *Myofascial Pain and Fibromyalgia*, ed. E.S. Rachlin (Boston: Mosby, 1994).
3. B. Edie, "Fibromyalgia: Cruel and Unusual," *Canadian Pharmaceutical Journal* 126 (1994): 500.
4. E. Vliet, *Screaming to be Heard* (New York: M. Evans and Company, Inc., 1995).
5. U.M. Anderberg et al., "Symptom Perception in Relation to Hormonal Status in Female Fibromyalgia Syndrome Patients," *Journal of Musculoskeletal Pain* 7 (1999): 21.
6. L.A. Aaron, M.M. Burke, and D. Buchwald, "Overlapping Conditions among Patients with Chronic Fatigue Syndrome, Fibromyalgia, and Temporomandibular Disorder," *Archives of Internal Medicine* 160 (January 24, 2000): 221.
7. E.W. Boland, "Psychogenic Rheumatism: The Musculoskeletal Expression of Psychoneurosis," *Annals of Rheumatoid Disorders* 6 (1947): 1947.
8. F. Wolfe et al., "The Prevalence and Characteristics of Fibromyalgia in the General Population," *Arthritis and Rheumatism* 38 (1995): 19.
9. M. Williamson, *Fibromyalgia: A Comprehensive Approach* (New York: Walker and Company, 1996).
10. M.B. Yunus, "Fibromyalgia Syndrome and Myofascial Pain Syndrome: Clinical Features, Laboratory Tests, Diagnosis, and Pathophysiologic Mechanisms," in *Myofascial Pain and Fibromyalgia*, ed. E.S. Rachlin (Boston: Mosby, 1994).
11. M. Williamson, *Fibromyalgia: A Comprehensive Approach* (New York: Walker and Company, 1996).
12. J.J. Luff, "The Various Forms of Fibrositis and Their Treatment," *British Medical Journal* 1 (1913): 756.
13. E.W. Boland, "Psychogenic Rheumatism: The Musculoskeletal Expression of Psychoneurosis," *Annals of Rheumatoid Disorders* 6 (1947): 1947.
14. H. Moldofsky et al., "Musculoskeletal Symptoms and Non-REM Sleep Disturbance in Patients with 'Fibrositis' Syndrome and Healthy Subjects," *Psychosomatic Medicine* 37 (1975): 341.

15. M.B. Yunus, A.T. Masi, J.J. Calabro et al., "Primary Fibromyalgia (Fibrositis): Clinical Study of 50 Patients with Matched Normal Controls," *Seminars in Arthritis and Rheumatism* 11 (1981): 151.
16. D. Goldenberg, "Fibromyalgia Syndrome: An Emerging but Controversial Condition," *JAMA* 257 (1987): 2802.
17. U. Mahring, "Fibromyalgia: Still No Silver Bullet," *Journal of the American Chiropractic Association* (2000): 30.
18. J.L. Rogers and S.J. Maurizio, "A Needs Assessment as a Basis for Health Promotion for Individuals with Fibromyalgia," *Family and Community Health* 22 (January 2000): 66.
19. Ibid.
20. T. Johnson, "Brain Surgery for Chronic Fatigue?" ABCNEWS.COM, March 10, 2000.
21. J. Joseph, "Fibromyalgia Patients Have Lower Blood Flow in Brain," ABC NEWS.com (http://abcnews.go.com/sections/living/DailyNews/fibromyalgia 980408.html, April 8, 2000).
22. G.L. Nicolson, M. Nasralla, J. Haier, R. Erwin, N.L. Nicolson, and R. Ngwenya, "Mycoplasmal infections in chronic illnesses: Fibromyalgia and Chronic Fatigue Syndromes, Gulf War Illness, HIV-AIDS and Rheumatoid Arthritis," *Med Sentinel* 4(1999): 172–176.
23. S. Hurwitz, "Bacteria Links Chronic Fatigue, Fibromyalgia and Gulf War Illness," www.AmericasDoctor.com (September 29, 1999).
24. M. Kossoff, "I Hurt All Over," *Psychology Today* 32 (May/June 1999): 42.
25. Ibid.
26. L.A. McKeown, "Fibromyalgia: Malfunctions in Two Key Body Systems May Contribute to Disorder," WebMD Medical News, WEBMD.COM, 1999.
27. NIH Research on Fibromyalgia, www.AmericasDoctor.com.
28. E. Wilson, "Fibromyalgia at an educational facility: Is there a link to indoor air quality?" *Journal of Environmental Health* 61 (May 1999): 20.
29. C. Lyddell and O.L. Meyers, "The Prevalence of Fibromyalgia in a South African Community," *Scandinavian Journal of Rheumatology* Supplement 8 (1992): 94; M. Nishikai, "Fibromyalgia in Japanese," *Journal of Rheumatology* 19 (1991): 110.
30. Y. Kimura, "Fibromyalgia Syndrome in Children and Adolescents," *The Journal of Musculoskeletal Medicine* 17 (March 2000): 142.
31. M.B. Yunus and A.T. Masi, "Juvenile Primary Fibromyalgia Syndrome: A Clinical Study of Thirty-three Patients and Matched Normal Controls," *Arthritis and Rheumatism* 28 (1985): 138.
32. P. Clark et al., "Prevalence of Fibromyalgia in Children: A Clinical Study of Mexican Children," *Journal of Rheumatology* 25 (1998): 2009.
33. S. Bowyer and P. Roettcher, "Pediatric Rheumatology Clinic Populations in the United States: Results of a 3-Year Survey," *Journal of Rheumatology* 23 (1996): 1968.
34. M.B. Yunus and A.T. Masi, "Juvenile Primary Fibromyalgia Syndrome: A Clinical Study of Thirty-three Patients and Matched Normal Controls," *Arthritis and Rheumatism* 28 (1985): 138.
35. S. Roizenblatt et al., "Fibromyalgia Syndrome: Clinical and Polysomnographic Aspects," *Journal of Rheumatology* 24 (1997): 529.
36. D. Buskila et al., "Fibromyalgia Syndrome in Children—An Outcome Study," *Journal of Rheumatology* 22 (1995): 525.

37. M. Mikklesson, "One Year Outcome of Preadolescents with Fibromyalgia," *Journal of Rheumatology* 25 (1999): 674.

38. M.B. Yunus and A.T. Masi, "Juvenile Primary Fibromyalgia Syndrome: A Clinical Study of Thirty-three Patients and Matched Normal Controls," *Arthritis and Rheumatism* 28 (1985): 138.

39. D.T. Felson and D.L Goldenberg, "The Natural History of Fibromyalgia," *Arthritis and Rheumatism* 29 (1986): 1522.

Chapter 2

1. "Health Care Professionals Teaming Up," *Fibromyalgia Network Newsletter* (October 1994): 4.

2. Duckett, "Fibromyalgia Common in Family Practice," *General Practitioner-Family Physician* 1 (May 1988): 30.

3. "Fibromyalgia Syndrome: A Patient's Guide," The Fibromyalgia Network, January 2001.

4. R. Sheppard, "Mysterious Malady," *Maclean's* 112 (March 15, 1999): 50.

5. Americasdoctor.com chatroom (November 2000).

6. J.L. Rogers and S.J. Maurizio, "A Needs Assessment as a Basis for Health Promotion for Individuals with Fibromyalgia," *Family and Community Health* 22 (January 2000): 66.

7. S. Blum, "Fibromyalgia Treatment Strategies with Steven Blum," WebMd.com (June 23, 2000).

8. D. Mann, "Mystery Maladies Pose Challenge for Doctors, Patients," WebMD Medical News, (http://my.webmd.com/content/article/1728.60829, August 29, 2000).

9. M. Kossoff, "I Hurt All Over," *Psychology Today* 32 (May/June 1999): 42.

10. J. Teitelbaum, *From Fatigued to Fantastic!* (Garden City Park, New York: Avery Publishing Group, 1996).

11. The CFIDS Association of America, Inc., "Understanding CFIDS," (www .cfids.org, 2000).

12. L.A. Aaron, M.M. Burke, and D. Buchwald, "Overlapping Conditions among Patients with Chronic Fatigue Syndrome, Fibromyalgia, and Temporomandibular Disorder," *Archives of Internal Medicine* 160 (January 24, 2000): 221.

13. K.P. White et al., "A Study of Fibromyalgia-Chronic Fatigue Syndrome (FM-CFS) Overlap in the General Population," Paper presented at the American College of Rheumatology Sixty-third Annual Scientific Meeting, San Diego, CA, November 14, 1999.

14. M.B. Yunus, "Fibromyalgia Syndrome and Myofascial Pain Syndrome: Clinical Features, Laboratory Tests, Diagnosis, and Pathophysiologic Mechanisms," in *Myofascial Pain and Fibromyalgia*, ed. E.S. Rachlin (Boston: Mosby, 1994).

15. D.J. Starlanyl and M.E.Copeland, *Fibromyalgia and Chronic Myofascial Pain Syndrome: A Survival Manual* (Oakland, CA: New Harbinger, 1996).

Chapter 3

1. M.B. Yunus, "Fibromyalgia Syndrome: Blueprint for a Reliable Diagnosis," *Consultant* 36 (June 1996): 1260.

2. I.J. Russell, "Elevated Cereprospinal Levels of Substance P in Patients with FMS," *Arthritis and Rheumatology* 37 (1994): 1593-1601.

3. M. Kossoff, "I Hurt All Over," *Psychology Today* 32 (May/June 1999): 42.

4. B. Edie, "Fibromyalgia: Cruel and Unusual," *Canadian Pharmaceutical Journal* 126 (1994): 500.

5. H.D. Moldofsky et al., "Musculoskeletal Symptoms and Non-REM Sleep Disturbance in Patients with Fibrositis Syndrome and Healthy Subjects," *Psychosomatic Medicine* 37 (1975): 341.

6. T. DiGeronimo, *Insomnia: 50 Essential Things to Do* (NY: Penguin Group, 1997)

7. M.B. Yunus et al., "Short Term Effects of Ibuprofen in Primary FMS," *Journal of Rheumatology* 16 (1989): 527.

8. R. Godfrey, "A Guide to the Understanding and Use of Tricyclic Antidepressants in the Overall Management of Fibromyalgia and Other Chronic Pain Syndromes." *Archives of Internal Medicine* 156 (May 27, 1996): 1047.

9. U.S. Library of Medicine, *NSAIDs* (http://www.nlm.nih.gov/medlineplus /druginfo/nsaids202789.html, August 23, 2000).

10. R. Sadovsky, "Considerations in the Management of Fibromyalgia," *American Family Physician* (May 1, 2000).

11. J. Potter, "Tectonic Changes in Disability Law," *Fibromyalgia Network Newsletter* (July 1999): 14.

12. Ibid.

13. M.B. Yunus, "Fibromyalgia Syndrome: Blueprint for a Reliable Diagnosis," *Consultant* 36 (June 1996): 1260.

14. U.S. Library of Medicine, *Ultram* (http://www.nlm.nih.gov/medlineplus/drug info/tramadolsystemic202789.html, August 23, 2000).

15. R. Sadovsky, "Considerations in the Management of Fibromyalgia," *American Family Physician* (May 1, 2000).

16. L.M. Arnold and P.E. Keck, "Antidepressant Treatment of Fibromyalgia: A Meta-analysis and Review," *Psychosomatics* 41 (2000): 104.

17. M.B. Yunus, "Fibromyalgia Syndrome: Blueprint for a Reliable Diagnosis," *Consultant* 36 (June 1996): 1260.

18. R. Scudds et al., "Improvement in Pain Responsiveness in Patients with FMS after Successful Treatment with Amitriptyline," *Journal of Rheumatology* 16 (1989): 98.

19. R. Godfrey, "A Guide to the Understanding and Use of Tricyclic Antidepressants in the Overall Management of Fibromyalgia and Other Chronic Pain Syndromes," *Archives of Internal Medicine* 156 (May 27, 1996): 1047.

20. U.S. Library of Medicine, *Anti-depressants* (http://www.nlm.nih.gov/medline plus/druginfo/antidepressantstricyclicsystem202055.html, August 23, 2000).

21. Ibid.

22. Ibid.

23. R. Celiker and Z.C. Anakara, "Comparison of Amitriptyline and Sertraline in the Treatment of Fibromyalgia Syndrome," paper presented at the American College of Rheumatology Sixty-fourth Annual Scientific Meeting, November 1, 2000.

24. R. Sadovsky, "Considerations in the Management of Fibromyalgia," *American Family Physician* (May 1, 2000).

25. "Health Care Professionals Teaming up," *Fibromyalgia Network Newsletter* (October 1994).

26. U.S. Library of Medicine, *Fluoxetine* (http://www.nlm.nih.gov/medlineplus /druginfo/fluoxetinesystemic202247.html, August 23, 2000).

27. W. Reynolds and H. Moldofsky, "The Effects of Cyclobenzaprine on Sleep Physiology and Symptoms in FMS," *Journal of Rheumatology* 18 (1991): 452.

28. U.S. Library of Medicine, *Baclofen (Systemic)* (http://www.nlm.nih.gov/medline plus/druginfo/baclofensystemic202080.html, August 23, 2000).

29. H.D. Moldofsky et al., "The Effect of Zolpidem in Patients with FMS," *Journal of Rheumatology* 23 (1996): 529-33.

30. Arthritis Foundation, *Fibromyalgia Syndrome* (Atlanta, Georgia: Arthritis Foundation: 1998).

31. "Opiods: Who Knows Best?" *Fibromyalgia Network Newsletter* (July 2000): 6.

32. Ibid., 9.

33. Ibid., 9.

34. U.S. Library of Medicine, *Narcotics* (http://www.nlm.nih.gov/medlineplus/drug-info/narcotics202180.html, August 23, 2000).

35. A. Bengtsson et al., "Primary FMS," *Scandinavian Journal of Rheumatology* 15 (1986): 340.

36. D.L. Goldenberg et al., "A Randomized Controlled Trial of Amitriptyline and Naproxen in the Treatment of Patients with FMS after Successful Treatment with Amitriptyline," *Journal of Rheumatology* 16 (1989): 98.

37. D.L. Goldenberg et al., "A Randomized, Double-blind Crossover Trial of Fluoxetine and Amitriptyline in the Treatment of FMS," *Arthritis Rheumaology* 39 (1996): 1852.

38. D.L. Goldenberg, et al., "A Randomized Controlled Trial of Amitriptyline and Naproxen in the Treatment of Patients with FMS after Successful Treatment with Amitriptyline," *Journal of Rheumatology* 16 (1989): 98.

Chapter 4

1. S.P. Buckelew et al., "Biofeedback/relaxation Training and Exercise Interventions for Fibromyalgia: A Prospective Trial," *Arthritis Care* 11(June 1998): 196.

2. R. R. Pratt, M. Pratt, S.N. Blair et al., "Physical activity and public health: a recommendation from the Centers for Disease Control and Prevention and the American College of Sports Medicine," *JAMA* 273(5) (1995): 402–407.

3. K.D. Jones et al., "A Randomized Controlled Study of Strength Training Versus Flexibility in Fibromyalgia," paper presented at the American College of Rheumatology Sixty-fourth Annual Scientific Meeting, November 1, 2000.

4. V.C. Valim et al., "Comparison of Aerobic Training and Flexibility Exercises for the Treatment of Fibromyalgia: A Randomized, Controlled Study," paper presented at the American College of Rheumatology Sixty-fourth Annual Scientific Meeting, October 31, 2000.

5. D.S. Rooks and C.B. Silverman, "A controlled Trial of Resistance Training, Cardiovascular and Flexibility Exercise on Fitness, Self-Efficacy and Functional Status in Women with Fibromyalgia," paper presented at the American College of Rheumatology Sixty-fourth Annual Scientific Meeting, November 1, 2000.

6. K. Mannerkorpi et al., "Pool Exercises Combined with Patient Education for Patients with Fibromyalgia Syndrome: A Six Month Follow-Up," paper presented at the American College of Rheumatology Sixty-fourth Annual Scientific Meeting, October 30, 2000.

7. S. Richards and D.L. Scott, "A Randomized Controlled Trial of Exercise Prescription for Fibromyalgia," paper presented at the American College of Rheumatology Sixty-fourth Annual Scientific Meeting, October 31, 2000.

8. S.E. Gowans et al., "Six Month and 1 year Followup of Fibromyalgia Patients Enrolled in a 23 Week Exercise Program," paper presented at the American College of Rheumatology Sixty-fourth Annual Scientific Meeting, October 31, 2000.

9. K. Giuffre, *The Care and Feeding of the Brain* (Franklin Lakes, New Jersey: Career Press, 1999).

Chapter 5

1. "It's Not All in Your Head—Depression vs. Fibromyalgia," (http://chronicfatigue .about.com/health/chronicfatigue/library/weekly/aa062100a.htm, June 21, 2000).
2. Ibid.
3. D. Schreiber-Servan, N.R. Kolb, and G. Tabas, "Somatizing Patients: Part I. Practical Diagnosis," *American Family Physician* 61 (2000): 1073.
4. Ibid.
5. M.B. Yunus, "Fibromyalgia Syndrome and Myofascial Pain Syndrome: Clinical Features, Laboratory Tests, Diagnosis, and Pathophysiologic Mechanisms," in *Myofascial Pain and Fibromyalgia*, ed. E.S. Rachlin (Boston: Mosby, 1994).
6. D.L. Goldenberg et al., "A Randomized Controlled Trial of Amitriptyline and Naproxen in the Treatment of Patients with FMS after Successful Treatment with Amitriptyline," *Journal of Rheumatology* 16 (1989): 98.
7. A. Gamsa, "Is Emotional Disturbance a Precipitator or a Consequence of Chronic Pain?" *Pain* 42 (August 1990): 183.
8. A. Okifuji, D. Turk, and J.J. Sherman, "Evaluation of the Relationship Between Depression and Fibromyalgia Syndrome: Why Aren't All Patients Depressed?" *The Journal of Rheumatology* 27 (2000): 212.
9. T.A. Ahles, M.B.Yunus, and A.T. Masi, "Is Chronic Pain a Variant of Depressive Disease?: The Case of Primary Fibromyalgia Syndrome," *Pain* 1 (April 29, 1987): 105.
10. J. Joseph, "Fibromyalgia Patients Have Lower Blood Flow in Brain," ABC NEWS.com (http://abcnews.go.com/sections/living/DailyNews/fibromyalgia 980408.html, April 8, 2000).
11 A. Okifuji, D. Turk, and J.J. Sherman, "Evaluation of the Relationship Between Depression and Fibromyalgia Syndrome: Why Aren't All Patients Depressed?" *The Journal of Rheumatology* 27 (2000): 212.
12. M. Castleman, "Depression in People with Chronic Illnesses," (www.depression .com/tools/health_library/coping/chronic.html, May 2000).
13. Ibid.
14. National Institutes of Mental Health, "If You're Over 65 and Feeling Depressed," NIH publication no. 95-4033 (http://www.nimh.nih.gov/publicat /over65.cfm, 1995).
15. C.S. Burckhardt et al., "Assessing Depression in Fibromyalgia Patients," *Arthritis Care and Research* 7 (March 1994): 35.
16. K.P. White and W. Nielson, "Cognitive Behavioral Treatment of Fibromyalgia Syndrome: A Follow-up Assessment," *Journal of Rheumatology* 22 (1995): 717.
17. B. Singh, B.M. Berman, and V.A. Hadhazy, "A Pilot Study of Cognitive Behavioral Therapy in Fibromyalgia," *Alternative Therapies* 4 (March 1998): 67.
18. L. Vanderhaeghe, "Fibromyalgia: The Invisible Illness," *Total Health* (http:// proqust.umi.com, March/April 2000).

Chapter 6

1. C.B. Silverman and D.S. Rooks, "Complementary and Alternative Medicine Use, Cost, Effectiveness and Disclosure in Persons with Fibromyalgia," paper

presented at the American College of Rheumatology Sixty-fourth Annual Scientific Meeting, November 1, 2000.

2. Ibid.

3. N. Flanigan-Ross, "Using Alternative Treatments," (webmd.com, Nov. 10, 1998).

4. M. Sandberg, T. Lundeberg, and B. Gerdle, "Manual Acupuncture in Fibromyalgia," *Journal of Musculoskeletal Pain* 7 (1999): 39.

5. K. Thorson, "Acupuncture: Is It for You?" *Fibromyalgia Network Newsletter* (January 2000): 9.

6. NIH Consensus Conference, "Acupuncture," *JAMA* (Nov. 4, 1998): 1518.

7. American Academy of Medical Acupuncture, *Frequently Asked Questions about Medical Acupuncture* (www.medicalacupuncture.org/acu_info/faqs.html).

8. J. Horstman, "Acupuncture," *Arthritis Today* (May-June 2000): 78.

9. Natural Medicine Collective, *The Natural Way of Healing Chronic Pain* (NY: Dell Publishing, 1995).

10. G. Hains and F. Hains, "A Combined Ischemic Compression and Spinal Manipulation in the Treatment of Fibromyalgia: A Preliminary Estimate of Dose and Efficacy," *Journal of Manipulative and Physiological Therapeutics* 23 (May 2000): 225.

11. K.L. Blunt, M.H. Rajwani, and R.C. Guerriero, "The Effectiveness of Chiropractic Management of Fibromyalgia Patients: A Pilot Study," *Journal of Manipulative and Physiological Therapeutics* 20 (July-Aug 1997): 389.

12. S. Ng, "Hair Calcium and Magnesium Levels in Patients with Fibromyalgia: A Case Center Study," *Journal of Manipulative and Physiological Therapeutics* 22 (Nov-Dec 1999): 586.

13. National Center for Homeopathy, "Introduction to Homeopathy," (www.homeopathic.org).

14. E. Greene, "Massage Therapy for Health and Fitness," (www.amtamassage.org/publication/massage.htm, 1997).

15. Ibid.

Chapter 7

1. P. Cowan, *American Chronic Pain Association Family Manual* (American Chronic Pain Association, 1998).

2. N.M. Hadler, "If You Have to Prove You are Ill, You Can't Get Well," *Spine* 21 (1996): 2397.

3. F. Wolfe, "Work and Disability Status of Persons with Fibromyalgia," *Journal of Rheumatology* 24 (1997): 1171.

4. J. Potter, "Tectonic Changes in Disability Law," *Fibromyalgia Network Newsletter* (July 1999): 14.

Chapter 8

1. F. Wolfe et al., "The Prevalence and Characteristics of Fibromyalgia in the General Population," *Arthritis and Rheumatism* 38 (1995): 19.

2. D. Goldenberg, "Fibromyalgia Syndrome A Decade Later," *Archive of Internal Medicine* 159 (1999): 777.

3. "Health Care Professionals Teaming Up," *Fibromyalgia Network Newsletter* (October 1994).

Glossary

ACR   American College of Rheumatology. The 1990 ACR criteria are used to diagnose fibromyalgia syndrome.

acupuncture   A form of Chinese holistic medicine, which involves piercing specific parts of the body with fine needles; can relieve pain symptoms.

American's with Disabilities Act (ADA)   U.S. law intended to help prevent discrimination against people with disabilities in the workplace.

adrenaline   A hormone released by the adrenal glands when the body senses eminent danger. It is sometimes called the fight-or-flight hormone.

"AIYH" syndrome   Acronym for "all in your head!"

alpha-EEG anomaly   A sleep disorder causing a state of partial wakefulness within sleep itself; commonly found in many people with fibromyalgia.

alpha sleep   Stage 1 sleep during which the body begins to enter into sleep but the brain is still somewhat active.

analgesic drugs   Pain relieving medication; any type ranging from over-the-counter aspirin to prescription narcotics.

antidepressant   Any chemical used to alleviate depression by restoring normal levels of neurotransmitters in the brain, especially serotonin.

arthritis   A disease caused by joint inflammation, joint damage, or infection.

behavior modification   Therapy designed to break negative behavior patterns such as drug taking, avoidance of activity, dependence on others, and preoccupation with pain. This therapy encourages and rewards the very opposite of these behaviors: responsibility, independence, activity, and the desire to free oneself from pain rather than be bound to it.

biofeedback   A method of teaching people how to modify their body's response to stress by providing them with visual and/or auditory evidence concerning a body function, such as temperature, muscle tension, and heartbeat.

central nervous system (CNS)   The brain and the spinal cord.

cervical spine   The top section of your spine or vertebrae located in your neck.

cervical stenosis   A condition in which the narrowing of the spinal canal in the neck leads to compression of the spinal cord.

Chiari malformation   A condition in which the cerebellum rests lower than normal and some of its tissue slips down to cause spinal cord compression.

chiropractic   A system of therapy which holds that disease results from a lack of normal nerve function and which employs manipulation and specific adjustment of body structures (as the spinal column).

chronic   Persisting for a lengthy period of time, often throughout a lifetime.

chronic fatigue syndrome (CFS)   A group of symptoms of unknown cause including fatigue, cognitive dysfunction, and sometimes fever that affect especially young adults between the ages of 20 and 40.

CNS   *See* central nervous system.

cognitive-behavioral therapy (CBT)   A type of psychological therapy that focuses on changing negative and/or non-coping thoughts and actions caused by persistent pain, repeated treatment failures, and the tendency of pain sufferers to focus their attention on their pain so intently that it comes to dominate their lives to the exclusion of other activities.

cognitive restructuring   Changing the way you think about your illness.

cognitive therapy   A therapy developed by American psychologist Aaron Beck in the late 1960s and based on the belief that people who think they can control their pain, who avoid thinking the worst about their condition, and who believe they are not severely disabled appear to function better than those who do not.

cortisol   Hormone secreted by the cortex of the adrenal gland that is important for regulation metabolism of fats, carbohydrates, sodium, potassium, and proteins.

delta sleep   Stage 4 slow-wave, deep sleep.

drug dependence   The situation in which there is a strong need to continue taking a drug either to prevent withdrawal effects or to obtain a desired effect.

drug tolerance   The situation in which an increasingly higher amount of a drug is needed to produce the same effects previously obtained at a lower dosage.

fibro fog   A term used to describe the cognitive impairments of fibromyalgia.

fibromyalgia   A widespread musculoskeletal pain and fatigue disorder for which the cause is still unknown.

fibrositis   The old name that referred to fibromyalgia syndrome.

flare   Time period when symptoms are at their worst.

FM   A common acronym for fibromyalgia.

FMS   A common acronym for fibromyalgia syndrome.

guaifenesin   A medication used to loosen and liquefy mucus. Sometimes used as an alternative treatment for fibromyalgia.

herb   A plant with a fleshy stem often used in seasoning or medications.

homeopathy   A system of medical treatment based on the use of small quantities of a substance that in larger doses produces symptoms similar to the disease being treated.

hydrotherapy   Treating ailments with the use of water, usually warm water.

insomnia   Having trouble falling asleep.

irritable bowel syndrome   A condition that is characterized by excess gas, abdominal pain, bloating, constipation alternating with diarrhea, and sometimes nausea, hyperacidity, and mucus in the stool. Very common in fibromyalgia.

living foods   Raw, uncooked foods that offer the health-promoting components of oxygen, bioelectricity, enzymes, and alkalinity not found in uncooked and unprocessed foods.

massage   Manipulation of tissues (as by rubbing, stroking, kneading, or tapping) with the hand or an instrument for therapeutic purposes.

muscle relaxants   Drugs that act on the central nervous system to treat muscle pain and tightness (including carisoprodol, diazepam, methocarbamol, baclofen).

myofascial pain syndrome (MPS)   A condition characterized by multiple trigger points in all parts of the body that have been present for at least six months.

narcotic analgesics   Drugs derived from opium or opium-like compounds with potent analgesic effects. Often used to relieve intense pain.

National Institutes of Health (NIH)   The biomedical research granting institution within the U.S. federal government.

neurotransmitters   Molecules released from nerve cells that carry chemical messages across the minute distance between two nerve cells and deliver them by binding to a receptor on the second nerve.

NIH   *See* National Institutes of Health.

nonsteroidal anti-inflammatory drugs (NSAIDs)   Drugs that reduce fever, pain and inflammation. They are available both over-the-counter (ibuprofen, naproxen) and by prescription (etodolac, oxaprozin).

NSAIDs   *See* nonsteroidal anti-inflammatory drugs.

occupational therapy   Can provide patients with assistance in making modifications to work and home environments.

opioids   Any narcotic that has opiate-like activities but is not derived from opium. They are analgesics and suppress both the perception of and reaction to pain.

pacing   A behavioral therapy that helps you find a balance between doing too much and not doing enough.

pain threshold   The point at which a person begins to feel a painful stimulus.

physical therapy   Treatment using exercise, heat, water, massage and other hands-on modalities.

restless legs syndrome   Burning, prickling, or uncomfortable sensations in the muscles of the legs which tend to occur at night in bed or during prolonged sitting such as in airplanes or in theaters.

REM sleep   Rapid eye movement sleep, also known as the dreaming stage of sleep that occurs most often towards the end of the night.

selective serotonin reuptake inhibitors (SSRIs)   A group of antidepressant medications that slow the reabsorption of the brain neurotransmitter serotonin to counter fatigue (including Prozac, Zoloft, and Luvox).

serotonin   An important chemical produced in the brain for aiding sleep and reducing pain.

somatization   Expression of symptoms for which there is no physical basis; symptoms are thought to be due to mental or emotional problems.

SSRI   *See* selective serotonin reuptake inhibitors.

substance P   Neurotransmitter that communicates pain signals in the CNS.

syndrome   A collection of signs and symptoms that occur together and constitute a particular disorder.

team treatment centers   Medical centers in which health care providers from a variety of disciplines pool their talents to give each person personalized diagnostic and treatment care.

tender points   Specific locations on the body that hurt intensely when pressed; used as a diagnostic tool for FMS.

tricyclic antidepressants   Medications that affect the symptoms of pain, fatigue and sleeplessness by acting on neurotransmitters such as serotonin, norepinephrine, and histamines in varying degrees.

trigger points   Painful areas of the body that, when pressed, can cause spasm in adjacent muscles or radiate pain to other regions that are served by the same nerves.

trigger point injections   Injections of medications (such as the local anesthetic lidocaine) into the tender spots of the muscles.

upper cervical adjustment   A chiropractic procedure that corrects the position of the top vertebrae, the atlas and/or axis.

Index

Aaron, Leslie A., 57, 58–59, 61
Acupuncture, 172, 174–178
Adler, Gail K., 27
Advil, 75, 76
Aerobic exercises, 120, 122, 128
Age at diagnosis, 30
Air quality, 28–29
Air temperature, 122
AIYH ("all in your head") syndrome, 141–146
Alpha-EEG anomaly, 74
Alternative medicine. *See* Complementary
    and alternative medicine (CAM)
Ambien (Zolpidem), 80, 87, 89, 111
American College of Rheumatology (ACR)
    diagnostic criteria, 8, 51, 54, 252
Americans with Disabilities Act (ADA),
    231, 232
Amitriptyline (Elavil and others), 80–81, 87,
    94, 95, 101, 117
Antidepressants
    for FMS symptoms, 78–79
    Karen's story, 84–86
    selective serotonin reuptake inhibitors
        (SSRIs), 82–84, 87
    tricyclic, 79–82, 83, 87, 89, 96
Arnica, 197
Arnold, Lesley M., 80
Arthritis
    as coexisting diagnosis, 2, 20, 41, 49, 50,
        63, 64
    comparison to fibromyalgia, 5, 9, 27, 30,
        31, 143, 148, 257
    complementary and alternative therapies
        for, 176, 181
    nonsteroidal anti-inflammatory drugs for,
        75, 76, 77
    warm-water exercises for, 127–128

Arthritis and Fibromyalgia Helpbook, 247
Ashendorf, Douglas, 109
Aspirin, 76, 187
Astin, John, 169, 207–208
Attitudes toward fibromyalgia patients
    changing, 267–269
    correct diagnosis and, 42–49
    doctors' viewpoints, 42–43
    somatization label, 143–145

Barsky, Arthur, 143
Bath, essential oil, 191–192
B-complex supplement, 190
Beck, Aaron, 159
Beck Depression Inventory, 152
Behavioral therapy
    goal setting, 167
    pacing, 165
    pain triggers and consequences, 162–164
    pleasurable activities, 166
    scheduled fun, 165–166
    sleep hygiene, 166–167
Belgrade, Miles, 175
Bennett, Robert, 78, 83, 90–91, 92, 260,
    265, 266
Benson, Herbert, 136
Biofeedback, 139–140
Blum, Steven, 43
Bohr, Thomas, 143
Boswellan cream, 191
Bourne, Leslie, 156, 157
Bowyer, S., 31
Bradley, Laurence, 57–58, 59, 60,
    150, 260
Breathing, deep, 125, 132–133
Buchwald, Debra, 38
Burckhardt, Carol S., 152, 266

Calcium and magnesium supplements, 191
Caldwell, David S., 54
Calms forte, 195–196
Carisoprodol (Soma), 86, 87, 88, 89
Cause(s), possible
   central nervous system disturbance,
     25–29
   current research on, 259–261
   genetic vulnerability, 18
   as medical riddle, 17
   mycoplasm bacterium, 24–25, 261
   spinal cord compression, 22–24, 261
   subset theory, 261–265
   theory testing and, 20–22
   triggers, 18–20
Celebrex, 77, 87
Celexa (citalopram), 82, 87, 99
Central nervous system disturbance
   altered pain perception, 26–27
   malfunction in CNS systems, 27–29
   as new research direction, 25–26
Central sensitivity syndromes (CSS), 62–64
Children
   fibromyalgia in, 30–33
   talking about your fibromyalgia to,
     223–227
Chiropractic treatment, 178–184
Chronic fatigue syndrome (CFS)
   as central sensitivity syndrome, 62–64
   mycoplasm bacterium and, 24
   symptoms, 16, 55–59
Clark, Sharon, 266
Clauw, Daniel, 18, 19, 22, 23, 25, 28, 42,
   260
Clement, Brian, 203, 205
Coenzyme Q$_{10}$, 210–211
Cognitive-behavioral therapy, 158–159
Cognitive therapy, 159–162
Communication with family
   general tips on, 220–223
   talking about symptoms, 219–220
   talking to children about fibromyalgia,
     223–227, 228
Complementary and alternative medicine
   (CAM)
   acupuncture, 172, 174–178
   chiropractic treatment, 178–184
   guaifenesin, 184–189
   herbs and supplements, 189–192, 208
   homeopathy, 192–198
   Maria's story, 208–211
   massage, 198–202, 204

   nutrition, 202–206
   plotting progress with, 172–173
   popularity of, 171, 172
   quackery, 206–208
   questions to ask practitioners, 173
Confusion, 6–8
Conn, Doyt, 2
Copeland, Mary Ellen, 60
Cortisol, 27–28, 129–130, 150, 157
Cowan, Penney, 217–220, 222, 249–250
Crofford, Leslie, 261

Dantrolene (Dantrium), 86, 87, 88
Deep breathing, 125, 132–133
Definition of fibromyalgia, 1
Delta sleep, 6, 72–73
Depression
   as coexisting diagnosis, 63
   organizations to contact, 153
   overlap dilemma, 151–153
   as separate illness, 146–151
   Stacie's story, 153–156
   as symptom, 8–9
Dexamethasone suppression test, 150
Diagnosis
   American College of Rheumatology
     (ACR) criteria, 8, 51, 54, 252
   bad news about, 37–38
   credibility problem, 38–41
   dangerous assumptions and, 64
   doctors and, 42–49, 254–256
   good news about, 37
   incomplete fibromyalgia, 54
   overlapping conditions, 55–64
   "ruling out" process, 49–51
   tender point sites used for, 51–53
Diet, 202–206
Disability, work
   controversy over, 237–241
   filing for, 241–244
Doctors
   changing attitudes of, 254–256
   finding the right doctor, 42–49
   somatization label from, 143–145
Dolorimeter, 52
Drugs. *See* Medications
Duffy, Kathleen, 189–192

Elavil (amitriptyline), 80–81, 87, 94, 95,
   101, 117
Epidemiology, 29–33, 252, 257
Epstein-Barr virus, 12, 13, 19

Exercise
  amount of, 125–127
  at-home, 119, 122–125, 126
  benefits of, 108–109
  cookie-cutter programs, 119
  importance of, 105–106
  instruction, 109
  pain-exercise cycle, 107
  personal stories regarding, 109–112,
     117–119, 127–128
  physical therapy, 112–119
  studies, 120–121
  warm-water, 127–128

Family life
  adjustments necessary in, 215–217
  communication tips, 220–223
  feelings of loved ones, 217–219
  successful treatment and, 213–215
  talking about symptoms and, 219–220
  talking to children about fibromyalgia,
     223–227, 228
Fatigue. See also Chronic fatigue syndrome;
     Treatment for fibromyalgia symptoms
  common drug-treatment options for, 87
  as primary symptom, 3, 5
  sleep disturbances and, 5–6, 19, 74
Ferguson, Ginger H., 11
Fibro fog, 6–8
Fibromalasia, 16
Fibromyalgia
  cause of, 17–29
  defined, 1
  diagnostic procedures, 51–53
  epidemiology, 29–33, 252, 257
  expected course of, 34–35
  history of, 13–17
  names given to, 16–17
  symptoms, 2–10
Fibromyalgia Network, 1, 41, 42–43, 45,
     237, 249, 257
Fibromyalgia Network Newsletter, 78, 175, 266
Fibrositis, 14, 15, 16
Flexeril (cyclobenzaprine), 86, 87, 88, 99, 111
Fun, scheduled, 165–166

Gaddy, Jennifer, 193–194
Gardner, Elliott, 91
Genetic vulnerability, 18
Gentle-motion exercises, 122–123
Gilbertson, Barbara, 176
Ginger, powdered, 190
Ginseng, 191
Giuffre, Ken, 69, 88, 106

Gleason, Rae, 254–255, 265, 267
Godfrey, Robert, 76, 81
Goldberg, Aileen, 187–189
Goldenberg, Don L., 15, 66, 95, 96
Gostine, Mark, 112
Greene, Elliot, 198
Greer, Jane, 227–230
Guaifenesin, 184–189

Hadler, N. M., 240
Hahnemann, Samuel, 192
Hamstring stretch, 124
Harris, Louella, 183–184
Harris, Richard, 183
Hartz, Arthur J., 43
Health insurance companies, 38–39,
     258–259. See also Work disability
Heffez, Dan S., 22, 23, 185, 260
Herbs and supplements, 189–192, 208
History of fibromyalgia, 13–17
Homeopathy, 192–198
Hormones
  cortisol, 27–28, 129–130, 150, 157
  melatonin, 96, 192, 198
  in women, 7, 27–28, 199
Horstman, Judith, 177

Ibuprofen, 76, 77, 87
Ignatia, 197
Imagery, 134–135, 172
Incomplete fibromyalgia, 54
Insurance companies, 38–39, 258–259. See
     also Work disability
Irritable bowel syndrome (IBS), 2, 8, 29, 62,
     63, 176

Juvenile primary fibromyalgia syndrome
     (JPFS), 30–33

Kali carb, 195
Kali phos, 195
Kennedy, Paddy, 136, 137, 139
Kimura, Yukiko, 30
Korn, Clifford, 200–202
Kossoff, Mirinda, 26
Kuprowski, Stefan, 170

Lachesis, 197
Lapp, Charles, 78
Leung, Frances, 42
Limomine, 198
Lioresal (baclofen), 86, 87, 88
Lorig, Kate, 247–249
Luff, A. J., 14
Lycopodium, 196

Mahring, Urscia, 15, 179–180
Marital problems, 213–219
Masi, A. T., 31, 33
Massage, 198–202, 204
Maurizio, S., 19
McCain, Glenn, 80, 158
Mease, Philip, 266
Medications
    antidepressants, 78–86, 87, 89
    cautious use of, 96–98
    chronic pain and, 68–70
    combination therapy, 94–96
    conditions accompanying fibromyalgia
        and, 100
    individualized approach to, 65–66
    muscle relaxants, 86–88, 89, 96
    narcotic analgesics, 87, 90–93, 96, 97
    nonsteroidal anti-inflammatory drugs
        (NSAIDs), 75–77, 87, 96
    Raylene's story, 100–103
    sleep disorders and, 70–74
    sleeping pills, 88–90
    trial and error process for, 98–103
    trigger point injections, 93–94
    Ultram, 77–78, 94, 96
Meditation, 136–139
Melatonin, 96, 192, 198
Menopause, 7, 199
Mental imagery, 134–135, 172
Methyl sulfonyl methane (MSM), 191
Mind-body connection
    AIYH ("all in your head") syndrome,
        141–146
    depression and fibromyalgia, 146–156
Mind-body therapy
    balance, 168–170
    behavioral therapy, 162–168
    cognitive-behavioral therapy, 158–159
    cognitive therapy, 159–162
    hope, 170
    pain cycle and, 156–157
    spiritual strength, 169
Moldofsky, Harvey, 70, 74, 86, 89
Morphine, 87, 90, 93, 215, 216
Muscle relaxants, 86–88, 89, 96
Muscles, reconditioning, 113–114
Myofascial pain syndrome (MPS)
    as central sensitivity syndrome,
        62–64
    defined, 59
    differences between fibromyalgia and, 55,
        59–62
    trigger-point injections for, 93–94

Nadler, Leslie, 162–166
Names given to fibromyalgia, 16–17
Narcotic analgesics, 87, 90–93, 96, 97
National Institutes of Health (NIH),
    256–257
National Organization for Social
    Security Claimant Representatives
    (NOSSCR), 244
Neck stretch, 124
Neurasthenia, 14
Neurotransmitters, 69–70, 74, 79, 175. *See
    also* Serotonin
Nicolson, Garth L., 24, 261
Nielson, W., 158
Nocioceptors, 69
Nongonococcal urethritis, 24
Nonsteroidal anti-inflammatory drugs
    (NSAIDs), 75–77, 96
Nutrition, 202–206

Okifuji, Akiko, 150
Olson, Jane, 261
Overlapping conditions
    central sensitivity syndromes, 62–64
    chronic fatigue syndrome, 55–59
    myofascial pain syndrome, 59–62

Pain. *See also* Treatment for fibromyalgia
        symptoms
    altered perception of, 26–27
    chronic, 68–70
    complementary and alternative therapies
        for, 173–211
    exercise and, 106–108, 127
    medication for, 74–103
    mind-body therapy for, 156–170
    negative thoughts and, 156–157
    as primary symptom, 3, 4
    relaxation for reducing, 130–131
    talking about, 220
    tender point sites, 51–53
Pain-exercise cycle, 107
Palmer, David Daniel, 178
Pamelor (nortriptyline), 80, 85, 87
Passive therapies, 113–114
Paxil (paroxetine), 82, 83, 85, 87, 94, 99, 149
Pedersen, Caron, 10, 12–13
Personal stories about fibromyalgia
    childhood fibromyalgia, 31–32
    complementary therapies, 208–211
    depression, 148–149, 153–156
    diagnosis, 39–41, 44–46
    exercise benefits, 109–112, 117–119,
        127–128

Personal stories about fibromyalgia,
    continued
    family life, 215–217, 225–227
    genetic role, 20
    good day/bad day roller-coaster, 34–35
    guaifenesin, 187–189
    living well, 249–250
    massage benefits, 200–201
    medications, 84–86, 97–98, 101–102
    Qi Gong meditation, 136–139
    relationship with yourself, 244–246
    sexuality, 230
    typical journey with fibromyalgia, 10,
        12–13
    upper cervical adjustment, 183–184
    work life, 232–237, 238–240
Pharmaceutical companies, 257–258
Phosphoric acid, 198
Physical therapy, 112–119
Physicians
    changing attitudes of, 254–256
    finding the right doctor, 42–49
    somatization label from, 143–145
Pilates, 210
Pleasurable activities, 166
Population with fibromyalgia, 29–33, 252
Postural training, 124–125
Preece, Cameron, 214–215
Progressive muscle relaxation, 135–136
Prozac (fluoxetine), 82, 83, 87, 95, 99
Psychogenic rheumatism, 14, 16

Qi, 174
Qi Gong meditation, 136–139
Quackery, 206–208

Race, 30
Randolph, Pat, 172
Relaxation
    for pain reduction, 130–131
    as a skill, 132
    stress response and, 128–130
Relaxation techniques
    deep breathing, 125, 132–133
    mental imagery, 134–135
    progressive muscle relaxation, 135–136
    Qi Gong meditation, 136–139
Research
    current, 259–261
    on exercise and fibromyalgia, 120–121
    on fibromyalgia in children, 30–31, 33
    first controlled study on clinical charac-
        teristics, 15
    funding for, 256–258

mycoplasm bacterium study, 24–25, 261
    new directions in, 25–29
    spinal compression study, 23–24, 261
Restless legs syndrome (RLS), 6, 10, 62, 90
Reynolds, John, 86
Rifkin, Arthur, 150
Rights, basic, 222
Rodgers, J., 19
Roettcher, P., 31
Rosner, Michael, 22, 23, 185, 261
Rowe, Peter, 260
Russell, Jon, 26, 27, 70, 251–254, 255, 256,
    258, 259–260

St. Armand, R. Paul, 184–187
Scherger, Joseph E., 39, 43, 46–48, 71, 103
Scheufele, Diane, 119, 122, 123, 124, 125
Selective serotonin reuptake inhibitors
    (SSRIs), 82–84, 87, 96
Self-talk, 244–246
Sensory motor training, 114
Serotonin, 26–27, 70, 74, 75, 77, 78, 79, 80,
    82, 95, 108, 175
Sexuality, 227–230
Sferra, Vincent, 86, 113–117
Siberian ginseng, 191
Sinequan (doxepin), 80, 87, 99
Singh, Betsy B., 158
Skullcap, 191
Sleep, poor. *See also* Treatment for
        fibromyalgia symptoms
    bath and tea remedy for, 191–192
    as cause or trigger for fibromyalgia, 19, 74
    drug treatment options for, 87, 88–90
    exercise and, 108
    explanation for, 70–74
    homeopathic remedy for, 195–196
    intensity of symptoms and, 34
    muscle relaxants and, 86
    as primary symptom, 3, 5–6
Sleep hygiene, 166–167
Sleeping pills, 87, 88–90
Social Security Disability (SSD) benefits,
    240, 241–244
Sohmer, Alec G., 242–243
Soma (carisoprodol), 86, 87, 88, 89
Somatization label, 143–145
Somatotropin, 74
Sonata (zaleplon), 87, 89
Spinal arch exercise, 123
Spinal cord compression, 22–24, 261
Spine-leg stretch, 123
Spiritual strength, 169
Stabilization training, 114

Starlanyl, Devin J., 60, 61
Staud, Roland, 260
Stiffness, 3, 4–5
Strength training, 120, 125
Stress
    avoiding, 140
    harmful effects of, 128–130
    muscle tension and, 131
    relaxation techniques for, 130–140
Stretching exercises, 123–124
Substance P, 26, 69–70, 175
Sulfur, 196
Support groups
    purpose of, 246–249
    tips for evaluating, 250
Support organizations, 259
Surveys
    diagnosis, 47, 63
    possible predisposing factors, 21
    symptoms, 11
    treatments, 67, 172
Symptoms, 2
    common primary, 3–6
    diagnosis and, 51–53
    expected course of disease, 34–35
    other common, 6–10
    weather and, 34, 122
Syndrome, fibromyalgia, 17

Team treatment centers, 265–267
Teitelbaum, Jacob, 55, 71
Temporomandibular joint disorder (TMJ),
    10, 32, 63, 181, 188
Tender point sites, 51–53
Thorson, Kristin, 257
Thorson, Steve, 34, 42, 237
Tizanidine (zanaflex), 86, 87
Tramadol (Ultram), 77–78, 94, 96
Trazodone (Desyrel), 79, 80, 99, 127
Treatment for fibromyalgia symptoms
    complementary and alternative treat-
        ments, 171–211
    exercise, 106–128
    individualized approach to, 65–67,
        261–265
    medication, 74–103
    mind-body healing techniques, 141–170
    relaxation, 128–140
    team treatment centers, 265–267

Trial and error process
    management of fibromyalgia with,
        98–100
    Raylene's story, 101–103
Tricyclic antidepressants, 79–82, 83, 87,
    89, 96
Trigger-point injections, 87, 93–94, 118
Trigger points of myofascial pain syndrome,
    59–61
Triggers for fibromyalgia, 18–20
Turk, Dennis, 231, 238, 263, 264
Turmeric, 190

Ultram (tramadol), 77–78, 94, 96
Upper cervical adjusting, 180–184

Vegetarian diet, 202–206
Vliet, Elizabeth, 7

Warm-water exercises, 127–128
Weather conditions, 34, 122
White, K. P., 158
Williamson, Miryam Ehrlich, 137–138
Willmarth, Eric, 131, 132, 134, 139
Wolfe, Frederick, 240
Women
    hormones and, 7, 27–28, 199
    incidence of fibromyalgia in, 29–30
    serotonin and, 27
Work disability
    controversy over, 237–241
    filing for, 241–244
Work life
    changing jobs, 233–234
    ergonomics, 232–233
    slower pace/less stress, 234–237
    to tell or not, 231–232

Young, Mark, 25
Yourself, relationship with, 244–246
Yunus, Muhammad B., 3, 9, 15, 31, 33, 37,
    48, 49–50, 52–53, 54, 59, 62–64, 66,
    76, 78, 80, 94, 142, 261

Zaleplon (Sonata), 87, 89
Zanaflex (Tizanidine), 86, 87
Zoloft (sertraline), 82, 83, 87, 127,
    146, 149
Zolpidem (Ambien), 80, 87, 89, 111

About the Author

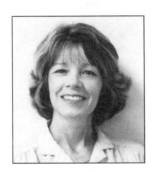 **Theresa Foy DiGeronimo, M.Ed.,** is a freelance writer who has written dozens of books on health, parenting, and communication. She is an adjunct professor of English at William Paterson University of New Jersey and lives in Hawthorne, New Jersey.

About the Medical Reviewer

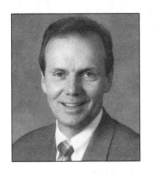 **Joseph E. Scherger, M.D., M.P.H.,** is dean of the College of Medicine at Florida State University, Tallahassee. He is the recipient of numerous awards, including Family Physician of the Year by the American Academy of Family Physicians in 1989 and Outstanding Clinical Instructor in the School of Medicine at the University of California, Davis, in 1984, 1989, and 1990. Dr. Scherger lectures frequently on fibromyalgia. He lives with his wife, Carol, and sons, Adrian and Gabriel, in Tallahassee, Florida.